More praise for
When the Air Hits Your Brain

"Dr. Frank Vertosick provides an amusing, insightful, and honest inside view of the training of the neurosurgeon. This highly readable account of daily life on the wards shows all the humility, fortitude, and humanity that genuinely underlie this sometimes not well understood but genuinely wonderful profession."
—DAVID W. ROBERTS, M.D.
Professor of surgery (neurosurgery)
Dartmouth Hitchcock Medical Center

"Well-told tales from the operating room by a thoughtful, almost humble neurosurgeon."
—*Kirkus Reviews*

"An engaging and refreshing book."
—*Booklist*

WHEN THE AIR HITS YOUR BRAIN

Frank Vertosick, Jr., M.D.

FAWCETT BOOKS • NEW YORK

A Fawcett Book
Published by The Ballantine Publishing Group
Copyright © 1996 by Frank T. Vertosick, Jr., M.D.

Fawcett and colophon are trademarks of Random House, Inc.

wv.w.ballantinebooks.com

Library of Congress Catalog Card Number: 96-91010

ISBN: 0-449-22713-8

This edition published by arrangement with W. W. Norton & Company, Inc.

First Ballantine Books Edition: June 1997

OPM   10   9   8   7

TO FRANK AND VERONICA,
who raised me to be whatever I wanted to be

Contents

Surgeons must be very careful
When they take their knife!
Underneath their fine incisions
Stirs the Culprit—*Life!*

—EMILY DICKINSON

I want to thank my wife and children for their support and understanding during the many long, dark nights spent writing. I also wish to acknowledge the many friends, patients, and colleagues who provided the inspiration for my stories. Finally, I wish to thank my agent, Victoria Pryor, and my editor, Ed Barber, for their willingness to listen to the ramblings of an obscure neurosurgeon.

Introduction

Neurosurgery is an arrogant occupation. Astronomers study the stars but never touch them. Particle physicists see God in the vapor trails of their great atom-smashers, but cannot see the particles themselves, cannot reach into protons and feel the quarks with their fingers. Molecular biologists sing the praises of the double helix, but the gene is forever an abstraction, invisible to the naked eye. These scientists must be content with the shadow nature casts upon their instruments and photographic emulsions. But not the neurosurgeon, for whom the greatest mystery of creation resides in a few pounds of greasy flesh and blood. Only the neurosurgeon dares to improve upon five billion years of evolution in a few hours.

The human brain. A trillion nerve cells storing electrical patterns more numerous than the water molecules of the world's oceans. The soul's tapestry lies woven in the brain's nerve threads. Delicate, inviolate, the brain floats serenely in a bone vault like the crown jewel of biology. What motivated the vast leap in intellectual horsepower between chimp and man? Between tree dweller and moon walker? Is the brain a gift from God, or simply the jackpot of a trillion rolls of DNA dice?

The answers to these questions rest at the uncharted

boundary between theology and science. We do know one certain thing about the brain: it is not unbreakable. When an unfortunate *homo erectus* plummeted from a cliff, suffering the first hominid head injury, mankind learned of the exquisite vulnerability of the pink goo between their ears. Surgeons of antiquity believed the brain sacrosanct, beyond their healing skills. As late as the nineteenth century, when bold surgeons attempted anything—even the repair of a beating heart—the nervous system was still considered off-limits. Although ancient shamans trephined holes in the skull to allow evil demons to escape, they knew that breaching the dura, the brain's leathery covering, meant the patient's sure demise from infection, bleeding, coma.

Some mornings I awaken and wonder how I ended up a neurosurgeon. One day I was a poor college student rummaging under my sofa cushions for a few quarters to buy french fries; the next thing I knew I was wrist-deep in someone's skull. What happened in between remains a blur.

There is a misconception that surgeons flock to their profession at an early age, drawn as if by a religious calling. Well, I didn't grow up planning to be a brain surgeon. I admit, as a child, I tried to build The Visible Head model—but I threw away the macabre plastic replica of a human noggin when the eyeballs fell out and rolled off the kitchen table. I should have taken this as an evil omen, but alas, I didn't. So here I am.

What draws people into "glamorous" medical careers? For some, it's vindication for being a loser early in life: the grade school wimp beaten in the playground, the high school geek who never had a date. For others, it's the secure (and large) income. As for me, I wandered too close to a dangerously seductive profession and wound up stuck for good, a fly in the spider's web. Had I never seen a brain operation, I doubt that the thought of doing brain surgery would have occurred to me. But once I viewed the living brain and was exposed to the seductiveness of the profession's arrogance in the flesh . . . I was hooked.

Brain surgeons have a well-cultivated public mystique, an aura of supreme intellectual and technical competence created by the imperious and brilliant Harvey Cushing, father of American neurosurgery and one of the first surgeons to specialize in brain operations. Cushing descended from a long line of medical men. Aristocratic and dashing, he drank his afternoon tea from fine china and stored his cigarettes in a sterling-silver case. He also had a keen eye for the media, fashioning himself into the medical superstar of the pre-television era—he even made the cover of *Time* magazine. Cushing knew that the brain was better PR than blocked colons and gangrenous legs. He endlessly exploited the public's fascination with his infant specialty.

But, in truth, the myth of the brain surgeon is largely that—a myth. While one can't be stupid and be a neurosurgeon, brain surgery isn't the most intellectually demanding occupation on earth. I can read a CT scan, but the people who designed and built the scanner's circuits tower over me in cognitive power. I see a blood clot crushing the life from a brain and deduce that the clot should be removed, but Gomer Pyle would reach the same conclusion.

My job is not easy, however. The high stakes make it tough. Unlike other parts of the body, the brain and spinal cord have little capacity for self-repair. If a general surgeon injures a piece of bowel during an abdominal operation, she simply stitches the injury, or, if that's not possible, removes the injured segment. With eight yards of bowel, there's plenty to spare. Even a trashed heart or liver is replaceable. But when I cut a nerve, it stays cut.

Neurosurgeons do things that cannot be undone. The grave consequences of our actions render even the most trivial of tasks difficult. Put a footwide wooden plank on the driveway and walk its length: no problem. But suspend that same board ten stories in the air and try walking its length again. The difficulty of a task transcends mere mechanics. Irreversibility of our missteps is one reason why I also awaken each morning wondering how I can get out of neurosurgery. The fly struggles in the web.

Our training period, simultaneously the worst and best part of our careers, remains one of the most arduous apprenticeships on earth. There are no neurosurgical prodigies. Little Elmo will never be the first in his advanced-track grade school to lop out a frontal lobe. Whether genius or dolt, everybody runs the same seventeen-year gauntlet from high school to board-certified brain surgeon. Why? Because neurosurgery, like all surgical fields, is a cult, a religion with mandatory rites of passage. All trainees must submit to the ordeal, must endure the withering years of death and disease, must feel abject humiliation at the hands of their professor-priests. In addition to professional brainwashing, the training process also achieves the unstated goal of turning out people who not only can *do* neurosurgery but also *look* like neurosurgeons in the Cushing mold: gray, chain-smoking males. The longer the program, the older and more persuasive the surgeon. A twenty-five-year-old man can pilot a spacecraft to the moon, but please keep him out of Mama's head.

This book details my odyssey into neurosurgery. However, the story focuses not upon my own talents, which are far from exceptional, nor upon any bizarre case histories or lurid physician behavior. No sex in linen closets here, no inside scoops on prominent medical personalities. The focus is upon the ordinary: ordinary patients and doctors facing difficult diseases and, at times, displaying extraordinary courage.

The book is a loose collection of clinical tales. I recall my residency as an anthology of patient experiences, not as a didactic education or a plotted story line. I remember nothing of the chapters on rheumatoid arthritis I read in medical school, but I do remember the distraught grandmother with gnarled fingers who could no longer roll cookie dough for her grandchildren. The book, like my training, is a collage of human beings.

The patient vignettes tend toward the gloomy side, and I may be accused of making the field of neurosurgery look like *Hamlet*, in that nearly everyone dies in the end. These stories do not mirror the field of neurosurgery at large, in which good outcomes vastly outnumber complications and deaths. I chose cases that became landmarks in my own progression from steelworker to surgeon of the central nervous system. Failure instructs better than success. A single death shapes the surgeon's psyche in a way that fifty "saves" cannot.

Neurosurgeons face terrible diseases—brain cancers, spinal cord injuries, head trauma, lethal hemorrhages. We confront patients deprived of speech, movement, vision. In many cases, disaster strikes them like lightning, in the form of sudden headaches, seizures, car accidents, or simple stairway tumbles. We see what no one would ever ask to see. Nevertheless, the nobility of the human spirit will always shine through the ugliness. The worst tragedies can be the most inspiring. During my training, I felt like Robert E. Lee, who, after witnessing great heroism in the midst of terrific carnage, mused: "It is well that war is so terrible, or we should grow too fond of it."

While based in reality, all of the names in this book have been changed and the true clinical stories altered substantially, even partially fictionalized, to protect the confidentiality of patients and the privacy of those who were and still are my friends and colleagues. The patients, physicians, and events depicted here are composites of many occurrences, people, and conversations that took place over ten years.

I did not intend to write with journalistic accuracy, or to chronicle my life, which after all is similar to the lives of a thousand other neurosurgeons. If my readers crawl into the mind of a generic neurosurgeon-in-training and witness what he witnessed, feel what he felt, fear what he feared—and marvel at the drama played out in any hospital, in any city, on any given day—then I have achieved my purpose.

1

The Rules of the Game

July 1. Neurosurgery residency.

Day one.

Five A.M.

A sickening wave of déjà vu flooded over me as I looked at the automatic doors to the "porch," the neurosurgical step-down unit. I had a sudden impulse to flee, to hide under my bed until it all went away. Six more grueling years of training loomed before me. Those years weighed heavily upon my brain that morning, like tons of ocean water submerging me, away from the sunlight of a normal life, normal job, normal things.

Before I could push the wall button to open the porch doors, they abruptly hissed apart on their own. There before me sat two men from my past: Gary, the hyperbolic smokestack of a junior neurosurgery resident who had ascended to become chief resident; and Eric, the once-jittery intern who was now a senior resident. I had worked with both of them years earlier, when I was a lowly medical student. We would be spending the next six months together on the boss's service, covering his pain patients as well as taking care of the trauma patients and other ER "hits" to neurosurgery. The "boss" was the chairman of neurological surgery, Dr. Abramowitz.

"Well, Eric, look who's arrived—Mr. Horner's sign himself," Gary said, referring to the clinical sign which had landed me in neurosurgery in the first place. Ancient history.

"Hello, Gary, you look—"

"Like hell, as always. Too much chocolate milk and nicotine—but, hey, whatever keeps you going? Listen, there isn't anything on the schedule this morning—the boss is testifying at a trial. Let's go back into the conference room. I need to spell out the rules of neurosurgery to you, from day one. After that, we'll take you down to see the Museum of Pain."

"The rules of neurosurgery? The 'Museum of Pain'?"

"Yeah, the rules. Rules you aren't going to read in any of the six volumes of Youmans' textbook. You'll see the Museum later—you have to see it to believe it." Youmans' was the bible of neurosurgery, the font of wisdom for trainees.

We went back to the small conference room where I would be making afternoon card rounds for many years to come. Gary went to the chalkboard and began to write.

"Rule number one: You ain't never the same when the air hits your brain. Yes, the good Lord bricked that sucker in pretty good, and for a reason. We're not supposed to play with it. The brain is sorta like a '66 Cadillac. You had to drop the engine in that thing just to change all eight spark plugs. It was built for performance, not for easy servicing."

"The patients seem to do all right," I protested.

"Yes, they usually do, but every once in a while something funny happens: someone's personality changes, a patient up and dies without warning—all little reminders that you are treading upon sacred soil. Which leads to rule number two: The only minor operation is one that someone else is doing. If you're doing it, it's major. Never forget that."

He took a sip of coffee and continued. "Rule number three applies equally well to the brain patients and to the spinal disc patients: If the patient isn't dead, you can always make him worse if you try hard enough. I've seen guys who have had two discs taken out of their backs and begged us for a third operation, saying that they had nothing to lose since they can't *possibly* be any worse than they are. So we do a third discectomy and prove them wrong."

Another sip. He went on. "Rule four: One look at the patient is better than a thousand phone calls from a nurse when you're trying to figure out why someone is going to shit. A corollary: When dealing with the staff guy after a patient goes sour, a terrible mistake made at the bedside will be better received than the most expert management rendered from the on-call-room bed or the residents' TV room. Look at the patient. Rule five: Operating on the wrong patient or doing the wrong side of the body makes for a very bad day—always ask the patient what side their pain is on, which leg hurts, which hand is numb. Always look at the films yourself and check that the name on the film matches the name on the chart. Always look at the consent and look at the patient's bracelet. To do otherwise is a setup for a *res ipsa*."

"Res ipsa?" I asked. "They never taught us that one in medical school."

"And they never will; it's a legal term. Short for *res ipsa loquitur*, or 'the thing which speaks for itself.' It means a malpractice case in which the error is so obvious that even a non-expert can see that a fuckup has occurred. A patient falls off the OR table. You cut off the left leg when it's the right one that's gangrenous. You send someone with a broken neck home from the ER with only an aspirin prescription. A patient bursts into flames during defibrillation. You take a disc out of a Mrs. A. Johnson when it was Mrs. J. Johnson who was supposed to have the operation. *Res ipsa* is checkbook time. Just write in a string of zeroes. Have I forgotten anything, Eric?"

Eric thought for a moment. "Well," he said, turning to me, "just remember the rules of any surgical residency: Never stand when you can be sitting, never sit when you can be lying down, never use the stairs when there are elevators, never be awake if you can be asleep, and always eat and shit at the first available opportunity." He thought some more. "And always agree with the boss. The boss *is* this residency program. When it comes to ego, neurosurgery is the major leagues, the NFL, the NBA. The big time. Grovel and beg at the appropriate times, and you'll do fine."

"This is residency now," Gary chimed in again, "you aren't the hotshot medical student or the know-nothing intern who can be forgiven any mistake. This is for keeps. This is your career. No more temporary rotations in pediatric endocrinology or tropical diseases. You'll do this shit until you die. Are you ready?! I said, are you READY!"

"Yes!"

Let the Games begin.

2

Slackers, Keeners, and Wild Cards

My descent into neurosurgery began in medical school, where I sought refuge from the real world. I took my undergraduate degree in theoretical physics—a great field if your name is Einstein. I was a steelworker, so my personality tended toward careers which offered me some realistic chance of making a living. The great Enrico Fermi, father of nuclear fission, once said that there are two types of physicists: the very best, and those who shouldn't be in the field at all. Any theoretician who isn't the best is a fraud, a pretender. I had done well in physics, but not well enough to pass Fermi's test. I decided, virtually by default, to become a doctor.

TV and movies foster many misconceptions about medical students, portraying them as drunken buffoons performing unspeakable acts with mummified body parts in anatomy labs, or as fully competent physicians (Judy can amputate the captain's leg! She's a medical student at Harvard!). In reality, medical students are glorified college students, people who think they know something, but don't.

Although a certain amount of rowdiness exists in any medical school, we were not picked for our social skills. I divided our freshman class into three groups. I was in the

12

biggest: the slackers, consisting of students who had garnered acceptable grades with a minimum of effort since
first grade. We studied only as much as absolutely necessary (and only at the last possible moment). We lurked in
the rear of the lecture halls, in the "prime bolt seats,"
from where an unobtrusive exit could be made if the lecture got too tedious or a good basketball game formed
outside. Most importantly, slackers never asked questions in class. Asking questions was a sign of weakness.

The second group, the keeners, were overachievers,
who hacked and bludgeoned their way to success through
work and more work. They planted themselves in the
front of the lecture hall, never exiting a class prematurely
even if diarrhea dribbled into their shoes. And they
always . . . ALWAYS . . . asked questions. A lecture on
the tying of shoelaces would still draw some keener into
the lecturer's face after class, waving a grade-school ring
binder and saying, "I didn't quite get it, the loop goes
under or over?"

The third group, the wild cards, entered medical
school because they knew someone, because one of their
parents had graduated from the school decades earlier, or
because someone on the admissions committee was
intrigued by an unusual entry on their résumés—"Spent
one year in Uganda ladling gruel into starving children."
Unfortunately, these admission criteria did not correlate
with IQ. The wild cards became our "cretin buffer," fat-
tening the grade curve for us slackers. The wild cards
never sat in the front *or* the back of the class—they never
went to class.

The first two years consisted of didactic lectures on
anatomy, physiology, pathology, and the like, with a few
brief contacts with patients thrown in as appetizers. The

real fun didn't begin until the third year. At that time, lectures ended and we were thrown into the hospital wards full-time.

Seven clinical tours of duty, or rotations, made up the third year: nine weeks of internal medicine, nine weeks of pediatrics, three weeks of anesthesiology, six weeks of general surgery, six weeks of obstetrics and gynecology, six weeks of psychiatry, and a three-week elective in the surgical subspecialty. My schedule arrived in August, listing my first rotation as the surgical subspecialty rotation. Great, I thought, I'll do cardiac surgery. Maybe I'll be a chest surgeon.

When I went to sign up, the secretary in the student affairs office dryly informed me that I could not do cardiac surgery, since the cardiac surgeons wouldn't let any medical students onto their service unless they had finished the six-week general surgery rotation first. She thrust a list of remaining possibilities at me: ear, nose and throat; orthopedics; plastic surgery; urology; neurosurgery.

Students were stacking up behind me. I had to think fast. Nose picking? Carpentry? Face-lifts? The stream team? The head crunchers? Nothing seemed as interesting as cardiac surgery. Oh well, it was just a crummy three weeks, anyway.

"Ahhhh . . . give me neurosurgery."

She jotted it down. "Vertosick, neurosurgery. Show up on the neuro floor, five-thirty A.M., September second. Next."

My fate was decided by a scheduling glitch.

Then it hit me: 5:30 A.M., as in before dawn? Was she joking?

On a gray September morning, I slogged to the hospital for my first day as a real doctor on the university neurosurgical service. I was about to step onto the slippery slope.

The neuro floor was dark and quiet, the nurses' station empty. I tracked down a nurse making his rounds and introduced myself, then asked him where I might find someone who would know what it was I was supposed to do.

"Look in the porch."

"The porch?" I had visions of some congenial place, full of wicker rocking chairs.

He pointed to a set of automatic double doors at the end of the long hallway. "You know, the porch, the neuro step-down unit . . . right there."

Thanking him, I wandered to the porch entrance. The doors carried the imposing label "Neurosurgical Continuous Care Unit, Authorized Personnel Only." I felt a bit of pride. For the first time in my life, I was "authorized personnel." I pushed a switch on the wall and the doors swiftly separated.

The porch was a small room with a tiny work desk at its center. Six patient beds, five of them occupied, were crammed in a semicircle around the desk. Electronic monitors dangled from the white ceiling and the walls were covered with metal baskets stuffed with gauze sponges, packages of gloves, IV kits, and other disposable medical paraphernalia. The air smelled of antiseptic. Faint monitor beeps were the only background noise. No wicker furniture here.

The patients, looking like giant Q-tips with their heads wrapped in bulky white bandages, were asleep (or comatose, I didn't know which). At the desk sat a thin, haggard man sporting a day's growth of beard and wearing a white jacket over his blue surgical scrubs. He hunched over a stack of charts, scribbling away. I tapped his shoulder and he jumped in his chair, startled by my intrusion.

"Jesus Christ," he hissed at me, "who are you?"

"Frank Vertosick, third-year student doing a neuro-surgery rotation. A nurse told me to come here. Is this the porch?"

"I'm Gary," he whispered back, calming down a bit, "junior resident . . . yeah, this is the porch. This is where we keep people who aren't sick enough for the intensive care unit, but are too sick to go out on the floor and be forgotten. Most of them are post-ops. Except that one."

He pointed to a young man, perhaps a teenager, with a thin plastic hose leading from his head bandages to a complicated contraption on a metal pole beside his bed.

"That guy's a head trauma. We're still watching his ICP, but he's wrecked. He'll go out to the graveyard until we can place him."

ICP, graveyard, place him. Clearly, the language we'd spoken in the first two years of medical school would be of little use here.

"ICP means intracranial pressure; the graveyard is the area of the floor where we keep the unconscious people; and when we say 'place him,' that means find some nursing home that will take him off our hands . . . he isn't going to be any better than he is now. I see you have a lot to learn."

"That's why I'm here," I beamed.

"No, you are here to be my fucking slave," he said with a broad grin. "Now, sit there like a good boy and let me finish my notes, then we'll get some breakfast."

Gary went back to leafing through the charts, jotting

down laboratory values and vital signs onto soiled note cards as he went. Every so often he would moan or mutter obscenities to himself, displeased with some chart entry. At last, he clapped the last chart shut, stacked the charts in a pile, and placed them in a basket for the porch secretary. He leaped from the chair and beckoned me to tag along. We exited the porch and took the long elevator ride down to the hospital cafeteria.

Gary broke the silence in the humming elevator as he lit a cigarette. "There are three residents and one intern on our service—me, the junior resident; Hank, the senior resident; and Carl, the chief resident. The interns float through on a monthly basis. Our intern right now is Eric Foreman, who's going to be one of the junior neurosurgery residents next year. We tend to ignore the interns, unless they're going into the program; then we kick the shit out of them. Everybody makes rounds in the morning on a different part of the service. Eric, since he knows nothing, rounds on the people out on the floor. They're generally pretty stable. I get the porch; Hank covers the intensive care unit; and Carl, as chief, gets to roll in at about six-thirty or seven. He doesn't see anybody in the morning; we just make 'card rounds' with him at breakfast, giving him a verbal report of what, if anything, happened at night."

"What'll I do?" I asked, still searching for what my role would be in this well-oiled machine.

"Well, after you get my coffee, I guess you should pitch in and help write progress notes on the patients on the floor. There are plenty of them and it's tough for Eric to get finished in time to go to the OR by seven-thirty. You see, every patient needs a progress note written on their chart every day . . . You haven't done any general surgery yet, have you?"

"Well, I haven't done anything, really."

Gary rolled his eyes. We exited the elevator and walked the short distance to the cafeteria. Loading up on corned beef hash and eggs, foods that hospital cafeterias serve in order to guarantee future admissions to the coronary care unit, I followed Gary like a lost dog over to a long table in the corner. Two other residents were already seated there, both dressed in street clothes.

"Carl, this is Frank, MS III." Gary addressed the more distinguished-looking resident, a slim man with a hint of white about his temples. "Frank's starting on neurosurgery this morning . . . No, wait, he's starting his goddamned medical career this morning!"

I shook the chief's hand.

"Welcome. This is Hank; he's a fourth-year resident." Carl motioned to the other resident seated beside him, a balding, portly fellow who waved at me and smiled as he continued to chew a large mouthful of food.

Gary and I took a seat and began to eat. Several minutes later, a frenetic figure darted to the table, his tray rattling in front of him, the coffee flying out of his cup. He had a boyish face and blond hair. This was clearly Eric, the intern, late for morning card rounds.

Carl cast a perturbed look at the intern, pulled his own stack of index cards from his lab coat pocket, and began the daily litany.

"Beckinger, room nine."

Eric flipped through his cards, locating Beckinger. I surmised that Beckinger was someone on the floor—Eric's responsibility.

"She's fine, afebrile, no headache, no face pain, wound is dry. She's now four days out from surgery."

"Has she pooped, yet?" Carl asked dryly, without looking away from his cards.

"Uh, I don't know."

"Well, goddamn it, find out. You know the staff man will go nuts if she hasn't shit four days out. Her fucking cerebellum could be hanging out of the wound and dragging on the floor, and he wouldn't care as long as her bowels are moving. If she hasn't done the deed, give her some mag citrate. . . . Rockingham, ten, by the window."

Eric was still scrawling "BM?=mag cit" on his Beckinger card. He hurriedly shuffled to the next one in his stack.

"Rockingham has some face pain, a little headache, temperature's 100.8, wound is dry. He's three days out."

"How much is a little headache?"

"Just . . . ummm . . . a little."

"Does he need a spinal tap?"

"I don't think so?"

"Did you wake him up, or is this what his nurse told you?"

Eric grimaced. "I didn't wake him, he looked so peaceful—"

"Chrissakes, Eric," Carl exploded, "you have to wake them up! I know it's early, but this isn't the Ritz. They can sleep at home, and I've got to know how they feel every morning. The staff guys will go around at eight this morning, the patients will start bitching that they were up all night and nobody's bothered to see them yet. That you stood outside the door and waved at them while they sawed logs isn't going to appease anybody. After breakfast, go upstairs and ask this guy how bad his headache is and come and tell me."

And so it went, patient after patient. First Eric, then Gary, then Hank. Each took his turn relating the patients. Eric and Gary took a ferocious beating, while Hank's presentations went unchallenged. Clearly, Carl looked at Hank as a colleague, while he looked at Gary and Eric as subordinates. He never looked at me at all. We finished at about seven-fifteen. Carl produced a large sheet of paper with the OR schedule for the week.

"Hank, craniotomy for meningioma, room twelve. . . . The only other case is one of the boss's face pain patients in room five. Gary and I will do that together. Eric, go back to the floor and take care of all the loose ends." The morning tribunal dispersed.

Gary took me over to the OR dressing room, where he gave me quick instructions on how to find scrub clothes and how to put on a hat, mask, and shoe covers. He also let me share his locker.

"Eric's being punished," Gary whispered to me as I changed my clothes. "He's not very up on things yet. Carl could have let him stand around with Hank on that brain tumor case, but he's been sentenced to the floor to be badgered by the nurses all day."

"What are you going to do?"

"Carl's going to teach me to open one of the face pain patients. I haven't done much more than help on that opening yet."

His face brightened. He was clearly looking forward to this. So far, I hadn't seen anything to get excited about— getting up before the trout fisherman, rounding on teenage boys who were headed for a nursing home,

eating greasy food, and watching grown men torment
one another.

Maybe seeing what went on in the OR would change
my mind.

I walked cautiously into operating room five, the first one
I had ever seen "in the flesh." Much smaller and less
grand than I imagined an OR to be, the room's walls
were covered with shiny green tile, the floor a hard,
blackish linoleum. The room had a cold and hollow feel,
like a large dormitory bathroom. Against the far wall, a
woman in full scrub dress shuffled metal instruments on
a large table. To my left, skull X rays dangled against
two light boxes hung at eye level. The patient occupied
the center of the room and was already anesthetized,
thick bore plastic tubing jutting from his mouth and nose,
the eyes taped shut.

Carl placed the man's head in a large C-clamp, and
then Gary, Carl, and the anesthesiologist flipped him
onto his right side and padded him with pillows and
pieces of blue foam rubber. They taped his body to the
OR table and fixed the C-clamped head to a contraption
at the top of the table. Gary quickly shaved a small patch
of the recumbent man's scalp just behind his left ear. The
two neurosurgical residents then exited the OR through a
back door. I hurriedly followed them, afraid to be left
alone in the OR. I feared I might commit some grievous
mistake—touch something, sneeze, fart, anything that
would ruin the operation.

The door opened into a smaller room almost entirely
filled by a long steel sink. Four faucets arched over the
sink like silver swans: the scrub area. The two men
taped their surgical masks to their faces, to prevent

fogging up the surgical microscope with their breath, and began to scrub their hands and fingernails meticulously. As they scrubbed, Carl swung around and spoke.

"Our chief of neurosurgery, Dr. Abramowitz, special-izes in treating pain patients. The man on the altar today"—(he motioned with a lathered finger to the OR door)—"has trigeminal neuralgia, also known as tic douloureux, or tic for short. Tic patients get sharp, stab-bing pains in their faces, sort of like a dentist drill hit-ting a nerve. What the boss—that's what we call Abramowitz—is doing today is the latest procedure for this condition. We'll drill a hole in the skull, find the trigeminal nerve to the face as it exits the base of the brain, and pad it from surrounding blood vessels using some bits of plastic sponge. It seems to relieve the pain without causing much numbness. The boss learned it from Jannetta himself, who pioneered this approach."

Gary and Carl backed into the OR, holding their drip-ping arms high in front of them. They dried their hands and gowned in dramatic fashion, aided by an OR assis-tant. After soaking the small patch of shaved scalp with a brown solution, Gary layered the prepped scalp areas with blue linen sheets until only the brown postage stamp of bald skin remained visible.

I stood, my back to the wall, while the surgeons huddled over that brown patch, slicing and dicing and filling the wound with dangling metal clamps, called "dandies," after Walter Dandy, another historical hero of brain surgery. The blue linen lining the brown patch stained purple with flowing blood. Buzzing noises and smoke filled the air as clamps cluttered the incision. Gathering my courage, I took a few steps closer to the table and peered at the wound. Beneath the pouting ruby lips of the mouthlike gash gleamed a broad white surface.

"Is that the skull?" I asked.

"Yup," answered Gary, "time for a drill."

A drill? Yikes.

At that moment a tall, craggy, white-haired man, about seventy years old, flung open the OR door and bellowed into the room, "How much longer, goddamn it? Jesus, Carl, how long have you been here? TEN MINUTES. I'll be back in TEN MINUTES."

"Yessir." Carl didn't look away from his work. "I was just showing Gary how to get through the occipital artery—."

"Great," the craggy man answered. "TEN MINUTES and I'm back. I want the cerebellum exposed by then." The door swung shut and the room fell quiet again.

I leaned over to Gary. "The boss?"

He glanced back over his shoulder. "None other."

"You heard the gentleman, we have TEN MINUTES to get into this guy's head," Carl barked. "Get the craniotome, Gary, and make a hole here, right behind the mastoid eminence."

Gary reached into a plastic pan and pulled out an instrument the size and shape of a flashlight. It was connected to a thick black hose which trailed down to the floor and over to a metal gas cylinder at the foot of the operating table. At the tip of the flashlight was a short steel cone topped with a spiral cutting edge.

"This is the craniotome; we use it to punch through the skull," explained Carl.

"How does it know when to stop before it plunges into the brain?" I asked.

"It has a pressure-activated clutch mechanism," Gary said as he pushed his finger against the tip of the conical drill bit. "When it penetrates the skull, the clutch disengages and the drill stops. Simple."

He squeezed the trigger on the craniotome and the drill whined to life. As Gary pressed the whirling bit against the ivory bone, Carl flooded the wound with water from a plastic syringe which could have been used for basting turkeys. Mounds of white bone chips flew from the deepening hole. Carl washed the bone dust onto the sheets. The whining continued for about a minute or so; then Gary's arm suddenly jerked forward, thrusting the still-running drill bit to the hilt into the skull. Quickly, the chalklike bone dust around the hole turned beet red. Gary reflexively pulled his finger away from the trigger and the drill stopped. The drill that was supposed to stop before it touched the brain had gone deeper than the residents had planned. A lot deeper.

"Oh SHIT!" cried Carl. "The fucking drill never stopped. Here we are talking about the clutch mechanism, and the thing doesn't shut off!" He grabbed the drill away from Gary and yanked it out of the patient's head. A torrent of blood and some stuff that looked like runny strawberry milkshake poured from the small hole in the bone.

"What'll we do?!" moaned Gary.

"WE don't do anything. YOU just stand there. Give me a Raney punch!" The scrub nurse handed Carl a large biting thing that looked like toe clippers from hell. He frantically tore at the skull bone, widening the small hole.

"I need to assess the damage, like real fast. Hopefully, we just trashed the cerebellar hemisphere . . . If we went down to the stem, we're all screwed." Carl's previous scholarly demeanor deteriorated to a nervous pratter. "I mean, God, I never saw a drill plunge so deep back here . . . Couldn't you tell you were going through the inner table of the skull? . . . Lordy, lordy, just so the stem is OK, tell me the stem is OK. . . ."

The door swung open. The boss again. "Is everything OK? . . . I SAID IS EVERYTHING OK?"

"Yeah . . . ah . . . fine, sir," Carl stuttered, "we just put a nick in the cerebellum, I think . . . We're fine—"

"FIVE MINUTES. A quick cup of coffee and I'll be in. In FIVE MINUTES."

Carl's gloved fingers twisted and turned instruments in the wound until at last he pronounced the drill's damage acceptable.

"It's just the lateral hemisphere. This guy's arm will be a little unsteady for a while, but he'll be OK. Give me a big cottonoid. The boss will never see it." He took a large white cloth square and covered the injury to the brain like a small boy covering a large scratch in the new coffee table with a newspaper.

I couldn't bear to watch any longer. I left, fearing the verbal explosion that might occur if the boss lifted up Carl's "newspaper." Given that "shit rolls downhill," I also realized that the lowest part of the terrain was me. Seeing Gary in the lounge after the case was done, I asked him how things had gone. He sat on a bench, still sweating and tremulous.

"Fine, I guess. The patient's fine, but, boy, I nearly killed that guy. I must have been leaning too hard on the drill or something, I don't know." He shrugged his shoulders and stuck out his left index finger. "You see this?"

"Yeah."

"That's about how big your coronary arteries need to be if you want to do brain surgery for a living."

Although I brought Gary coffee each morning, I was really Eric's slave for the remainder of my neurosurgery clerkship. Eric had more work to do, work that even a third-year student could do. The frazzled intern quickly taught me to remove skin sutures and change dressings. He dispatched me to ask patients questions he had neglected: What were their allergies, did they bring their X rays, had they had their morning bowel movements? I became the "scut doggie," rounding up laboratory reports, photocopying journal articles, fetching lab coats left behind in patients' rooms.

My real contribution was my slew of "H & P's," short for histories and physicals. The history consists of the patient's story told in his or her own words, and includes the chief complaint ("My face hurts when I eat"); the present history ("My face pain started three years ago, and has gotten worse since December . . ."); past history ("I am diabetic and have had my gallbladder removed"); current medications; allergies; occupation; smoking and drinking behavior; and so on. The physical is the physical examination. Even in an age of increasing technology, a patient's illness can be diagnosed over three-quarters of the time by the H & P alone.

Every patient admitted to the hospital must have an H & P written on the chart. On a busy day, the neurosurgical service admitted twelve or more people. Even an uncomplicated H & P took thirty minutes to perform, and the task of getting them all done before nightfall was daunting. Only Gary and Eric did H & P's; the senior and chief residents considered them menial chores. Gary lived in the OR, leaving Eric saddled with six to twelve hours of H & P's a day. Taught the fundamentals of history taking and physical examination in our second year, any third-year student could do a passable H & P. I became an H & P machine, cranking out four to six every day.

Of course, nobody read them. Clinical decisions did not turn upon my findings. The attending surgeon, having performed a very directed history and physical in the office, made the required decisions after some careful thought long before the patient ended up in a hospital. My H & P's were essentially bureaucratic exercises. With one fateful exception.

Harvey Rathman, a man in his late fifties, was admitted for the removal of a herniated cervical disc in his neck. His "chief complaint" was right-arm pain, increasing in severity over several weeks. Physical therapy had proved ineffective, and he now ate narcotics just to sleep at night. At an outside hospital, Mr. Rathman had undergone a myelogram: thick dye was injected into his neck to visualize the shadowy outlines of his spinal nerves on X-ray films. The test had disclosed that one of his neck's discs, the fibrous pillows between the vertebrae, had ruptured, "pinching" a nerve between a disc fragment and the bony spine.

While totally incapable of interpreting the X-ray pictures myself, I managed to find the printed radiology report which accompanied the patient's file. At the bottom of the report, it read: "Impression: small central to left-sided disc herniation, C56." Left-sided? But the patient's arm pain was on the right. How does a pinched nerve to the left arm cause pain in the right arm? I showed this paradox to Eric, who shrugged it off. He said

that misprints occurred frequently, and that the staff surgeon must know that the disc had really ruptured to the
right side or he wouldn't have brought him in for
surgery. "The radiologist probably just goofed up when
dictating the report."

I accepted this explanation and strolled down the hall
to see Mr. Rathman. It was nine in the evening when I
entered the dark room. Mr. Rathman sat in his bed, his
gaunt, lined face betraying his discomfort. He managed a
contorted smile and said in the hoarse voice of a career
cigarette user, "May I help you?"

"I'm Frank Vertosick, Mr. Rathman." I extended my
hand, but he declined to raise his ailing arm and simply
waved with his left hand. "I need to ask you some
questions and do a brief examination, for the record.
Now . . ." My voice trailed off.

"Is something wrong?" the man asked.

Something *was* wrong. As I glanced closely at his
face, it struck me that his pupils were grossly asymmet-
rical. The right pupil was tiny, but the left pupil was
huge, saucerlike. What was going on here? In an instant,
a flash of insight burst into my head from nowhere. Deep
in the recesses of my memory, brain demons below the
level of my consciousness pieced together the man's
diagnosis from the disjointed bits of knowledge garnered
during my first two years of medical school. The arm
pain . . . the smoker's rasp . . . the thin face . . . the
unequal pupils . . . it all crystallized for me in a rush. This
man did not have a ruptured disc! I stood over him,
frozen by the thought that only I knew what was causing
his arm pain. But I couldn't say anything to him. That
was not my place.

"No, nothing's wrong. Now, tell me about your pain

. . . when did it start?" So it went. I finished the H & P, thanked him, and left. I immediately grabbed Gary, who had just come out of the OR from a head trauma case.

"Gary," I said, breathless, "that guy, Rathman, in room fifteen, he's here for a cervical discectomy, but his disc is on the wrong side! And he has a Horner's sign! Go look for yourself!"

"What guy? What the hell are you talking about? You're babbling. It's ten o'clock. Go home." He bolted down a carton of chocolate milk and walked away. I chased after him.

"No, wait, I'm telling you that this guy is on the OR schedule for seven-thirty tomorrow morning and it's all wrong. He has a Horner's sign; you don't get that from a disc. Just go and look at him."

The iris functions like a camera diaphragm, limiting the amount of light entering the eye. Powered by small muscles, the iris becomes paralyzed if its nerve supply fails. If the iris is paralyzed, the pupil remains small. In bright light, when the normal pupil constricts to the same size as a paralyzed iris, the abnormality can be masked. In dim light, however, the normal iris dilates while the paralyzed pupil remains small—an asymmetry known as the Horner's sign. The difference between the paralyzed and normal iris is so pronounced that even a novice like myself could see it in dim light. When the staff surgeon had examined Mr. Rathman in a bright examination room, the Horner's sign was not there.

The nerves to the iris don't come from the cervical, or neck, nerves, but from the upper chest. This sounds bizarre—eye nerves coming from the chest—but the human body's blueprints can be hard to decipher at times. Mr. Rathman's C56 disc wasn't causing his pupillary asymmetry. Something was going on deep in his chest, gnawing at the nerves to his right arm and amputating the iris nerves. In a middle-aged smoker, the most likely explanation was also the most grim: lung cancer.

Gary paused. "Didn't he have a pre-op chest X ray?"

"Yes, it was read as bilateral apical pleural thickening."

"Hmmm, I guess a Pancoast tumor could be hiding at the apex under that pleural thickening and be missed on routine X ray," he muttered, almost to himself. "Well, let's have a look." He walked down the corridor to the patient's room.

Mr. Rathman, medicated with morphine, dozed as we entered. Gary gently shook him awake. The junior resident grasped the drowsy man's chin and turned his head left and right, squinting to see his pupils in the low light.

"I'm sorry, Mr. Rathman, go back to sleep."

Gary walked sullenly to the nurses' station without saying another word. He sat in a chair by a ward phone, reached into his pocket, and produced a portable phone directory. After finding a number, he punched the buttons and waited for an answer.

"Hello? Is Dr. Atkins in? . . . Dr. Atkins, Gary from the hospital . . . Listen, sorry to bother you, but this Rathman guy you have on for tomorrow, did you know he has a Horner's sign on the right . . . No, it's pretty obvious . . . uh-huh . . . Yeah, a Pancoast tumor is a real possibility. Sure . . . no, don't thank me, it was the medical stud who found it. . . . OK, so long."

He hung up the phone and grabbed the patient's chart, opening to a physician's order sheet. He wrote:

"Cancel OR. Polytomography of the right apex of lung in A.M."

Gary looked up at me with a stern face. "That's the easy part. The hard part is explaining to him why we are canceling his surgery." He got up and began the walk down the corridor again, this time more slowly. "I'll take care of it, Frank, that's why they pay me. Go home."

He didn't need to tell me twice.

Mr. Rathman's lung studies showed the expected crab-like growth at the tip of his right lung, a Pancoast lesion. A needle biopsy confirmed a squamous-cell lung carci-noma. No thought was given to removing it; his arm pain and Horner's sign were proof that the tumor had escaped his lung and was encasing his brachial plexus, the network of nerves in the shoulder. There was no hope of cutting it out now. He was transferred to the oncology service for radiation therapy. I never saw him again.

Mr. Rathman's case came back to me several months later, after I had left the neurosurgery service and was on my internal medicine rotation at the Veterans Hospital. I received a message that Dr. Abramowitz wanted to see me in his office.

At the appointed time, I was escorted by a secretary into the boss's lavish office. The walls were filled with diplomas, citations, awards, and autographed pictures of previous teachers and residents. He glared at me over reading glasses slung low over his long nose, his feet propped up on the broad desk.

"Please sit down."

I complied, almost vanishing into a plush chair. The boss bolted up and continued.

"I understand that you picked up a lung tumor in one of my staff men's patients, a man who was headed for a discectomy the next morning?"

"I just saw his Horner's sign, that's all. It was obvious because it was so dark ... it could easily have been missed during the day, a fluke really." I was nervous. Was this some sort of investigation of his attending surgeon?

"Still, you saved him an operation. Listen, we need good men for this program. How would you like a job when you graduate?"

"Doing what?"

He laughed. "Doing this. Neurosurgery. Becoming one of us. It's tough, but this is one of the best programs in the country, which means in the world."

I was stunned. "I'll have to think about it, sir."

"Well, don't think too long. Over one hundred people apply for the two spots we offer each year, and we like to pick them several years in advance."

Thanking him, I beat a hasty retreat. This was an honor, being offered a position in a premier program by an internationally renowned surgeon. But something bothered me: If this was such an honor, then why offer it to someone who got lucky on one patient? I remembered Groucho Marx's comment about not wanting to belong to any country club foolish enough to take him as a member.

And why several years in advance? I thought back to my grade school friend David, who committed to the seminary when he was only fourteen years old. Maybe surgical residency was like the priesthood: get 'em early, before they know what's happening.

At least David wised up. He now has three children and sells insurance.

3

Thanks for Everything

I was in the middle of my third-year rotation in medicine when the boss offered to make me "one of them." The medicine rotation, or clerkship, was offered at the local Veterans Administration Hospital, more commonly known as the V.A. (Vee-Ay), the Vah, or, more sarcastically, the Vah-spa—although it was hardly spa-like. Nestled behind the university football stadium, the V.A. looked like any 1950s-era federal building: bland and boxy, with smooth, yellow-brick walls tinged with industrial soot.

Our V.A. was one of the better veterans' facilities in the country. Most of its employees tried hard to do a good job, but the unmistakable footprint of government bureaucracy was everywhere: nowhere to park (unless you were one of the administrators), oppressive paperwork, outdated equipment. Management teemed with career drones who knew they couldn't be fired and acted accordingly. Surprisingly, the hospital's many inefficiencies didn't stem from a lack of money, since the V.A. was well funded. Regulations strangled the place, not poverty.

The V.A. holds fond memories for me. For medical students and residents, that musty building was, for all of its problems, a fun house filled with discussions of medical esoterica over cold pizza at three in the morning. A place for poring through hospital charts that stood taller than the patients. A place where a baby-faced third-year student like myself could be introduced as "doctor" without being laughed at. The hours were long, the supervision scant, and the aggravations many; but the daily struggle to provide quality health care to men and women who had served their country was rewarding. With the monolithic government as our common enemy, the V.A. forged personal bonds among the resident corps (also called "house staff"), often lasting a lifetime. Jim, my assigned intern-mentor during the third-year medicine rotation, remains one of my closest friends almost two decades later.

The public uses the word "medicine" in the generic sense to encompass all aspects of health care, from dermatology to orthopedic surgery to pediatrics. To the layperson, anyone with an M.D. is "in medicine." To a physician, a person "in medicine" is an internist—as opposed to a surgeon, radiologist, or psychiatrist. Internal medicine residencies train physicians to handle the non-surgical health problems of adults, such as diabetes, hypertension, and pneumonia.

During those crucial nine weeks at the V.A., I learned many of the minor technical aspects of being a physician: drawing blood, looking at X rays, interpreting electrocardiograms, writing orders. I hungered for this experience. The neurosurgery elective hadn't afforded any opportunity to do much beyond yanking stitches and percussing chests. The medicine rotation introduced me to the awesome authority invested in physicians: the power to violate another human being—legally. License to stick our gloved fingers into the rectums of humanity, to jam needles into spines, to thread garden hoses into colons.

I first tasted this intoxicating authority in my second week at the V.A. Jim, my intern, handed me a naso-gastric tube, together with a foil packet of K-Y jelly, and told me to insert the plastic snake into one of his cirrhosis patients in the big ward. The patient, nauseated from a bowel impaction, needed the tube to decompress his stomach and make him more comfortable (if having a half-inch tube in your nose is more comfortable than minor queasiness).

"You've seen me do it a dozen times," Jim reassured me as he dashed off to morning report. "Just stick it up his nose until you see it in the back of his mouth, then tell him to swallow. . . . When he does, just feed it in quickly. After about two feet are in, blow some air into the tube with a fifty-cc syringe and listen for the bubbles in his stomach with a stethoscope. That way you know you're in his stomach and not his right bronchus."

I nodded and went to the ward, my heart pounding and palms sweating. The V.A. still gets away with putting ten to twenty patients into a single large ward with beds separated by flimsy curtains. Private hospitals, on the other hand, typically allow only two patients in a room, and many newer hospitals have only single rooms. At the V.A., however, the older veterans preferred the compan-ionship of the ward and demanded to be put there, so there were few complaints.

I found my target propped up in his bed, his abdomen distended and a blue emesis basin in his hand. An elderly, rotund man with a bulbous nose and rosy cheeks sprinkled with thin, spidery veins, he smiled cordially. We talked for a bit; he had a soft trace of a southern accent, betraying his boyhood in Georgia. He rambled on about his experiences in World War II, when he was a bomber pilot flying missions over Berlin. Lifting his gnarled hand, he offered up a steel ring adorned with tiny wings as proof of his exploits, as if he knew that his bloated appearance was too removed from the trim, leather-jacketed aviator for anyone to believe him. Alas, almost forty years had passed since Berlin, and the war hero was now a retired peach farmer with a bum liver.

The tube insertion went badly. I couldn't get the damned thing up his right nostril. I tried the left nostril. That didn't work either, so I went back to the right side again. By this time the left nostril was bleeding profusely, rivulets of blood running down the patient's face into his mouth and onto his green pajamas.

The tube finally slithered up the nose and down the farmer's throat. Before I could say "Swallow," he gagged violently and vomited on both of us. The far end of the tube flew out of his mouth, even as the other end remained jutting from his nose. Horrified, I harshly yanked out the tube, as if I were trying to pull-start an outboard motor in his sinuses. He yelped—and then his right nostril started to bleed as well. I fetched paper towels from a nearby sink, wetted them, and spent ten minutes stanching the bleeding and cleaning him up as best I could.

"I'm terribly sorry; we'll try this again later," I apologized weakly, fearing his well-deserved anger at my incompetence.

But he just sniffled and smiled. "OK, Doc . . . thanks for everything."

After almost running from the ward, I stood in the hallway to compose myself. What had just happened to this man? A total stranger had walked up to him and rammed a weapon up his nose until he was bleeding like Old Faithful, halting the torture only after he had blown lunch all over himself in full view of six other patients on the ward. On the street, this would not be called a medical procedure, but assault and battery—with witnesses, no less! And, amazingly enough, he was thankful. Thankful! For "everything."

I glanced down at my white coat. This could not be ordinary clothing, I thought, it must be some sorcerer's cloak, this white linen, my only credential. It had not only shielded me from the ire of this combat veteran, but inspired his gratitude as well.

In the years that followed, I would do worse things to a human body than make it puke or give it a bloody nose— a lot worse. Nevertheless, another milestone had passed. As I threw away the nasogastric tube caked with bloody jelly, I felt the first inkling of what being a doctor involved. The intoxicant of power.

I wasn't sure I liked it.

All television medical dramas contain at least one "cardiac arrest." A dying patient being shocked, pounded, and probed by grim-faced professionals has been replayed so frequently in entertainment venues that the average layperson could probably manage a cardiac arrest just by having watched TV.

During my residency, I moonlighted in urban emergency rooms. As I resuscitated a heart attack victim in the ER hallway one night, another patient came up to me, pointed to my expiring patient, and asked if I had tried intracardiac epinephrine yet. I curtly told him to mind his own business and sent him to his own ER cubicle, then promptly loaded up the intracardiac syringe and followed his advice. The patient lived. Thank God for television.

Every hospital has its own method of announcing a cardiac arrest in progress. "Code blue" is a popular prime-time choice, but our hospitals used "Condition A," "Blue alert," or "Calling Dr. White." The operator's disembodied voice cried from every speaker: "Calling Dr. White, room 4835," and the code team dashed madly to room 4835, life support equipment in tow.

These encrypted messages supposedly avoided panicking the patient's relatives (even when they *should* panic). "Dr. White" is being asked to go to room 4835—no big deal.

In reality, euphemisms such as "Calling Dr. White" did little to alleviate public distress. Imagine the bustling lunchtime cafeteria of a busy urban hospital. The operator, who has been calmly reciting phone pages for the past hour ("Dr. Nelson, call extension 5545. . . . Dr. Rosenbloom, call the emergency room, please . . .") suddenly screams, "CALLING DR. WHITE, OUTPATIENT SURGERY" three times in quick succession, causing a dozen doctors to drop their forks midmouthful, bolt their lunch trays, and run away clutching metal boxes full of equipment.

The "Dr. White" phrase had one comical side effect. In the university hospital one morning, we had five "Dr. Whites" called in less than three hours. We thought the worst had passed when a sixth "Dr. White" directed us to a private room on the ninth floor. Rushing to the room, we found a very aged but otherwise quite robust-looking gentleman reading the *Wall Street Journal* and sipping coffee.

"Who called a cardiac arrest here?" angrily demanded the senior medical resident on the resuscitation team.

"I didn't call any cardiac arrest, young man; I simply asked the operator to send Dr. White to my room. My own internist isn't worth a damn and people have been calling for this Dr. White character all morning. I felt he must be pretty damned good if he's in so much demand."

Thankfully, the V.A. had no public-address system. The operator merely summoned the designated arrest team through their beepers. As a third-year student on the medicine rotation, I was assigned to the arrest team for the evening every other night. The team consisted of the senior medical resident, Kate; my intern, Jim; a fourth-year student, Pam; and me. At least once a night we answered the call of our whining arrest beepers. We would run a dozen flights of stairs to the designated location and arrive to find some unfortunate soul who had, in euphemistic hospital lingo, CTB'd, or "ceased to breathe." The poor souls always had a damned good reason for "ceasing to breathe," like being riddled with cancer or being older than the Appalachians, but we were called anyway.

Before proceeding with resuscitation, Kate would glance through her sign-out sheet to see which patients were marked with the letters DNR—do not resuscitate. At that time, living wills and frank discussions with patients about life support were much less common than they have become in recent years, and so we had to initiate some effort to revive a hopeless case. The floor nurses wheeled in the big red "crash cart" containing the defibrillator and drugs, I would hook up the EKG monitor, Pam would draw blood, and Kate would place an endotracheal tube. The three junior people took turns "bagging" oxygen into the patient's lungs with a big green balloon, the Ambu bag, while Kate barked out commands. We conned one of the orderlies or respiratory therapists into doing the exhausting manual chest compressions, which are supposed to squeeze blood from the motionless heart.

Despite witnessing dozens of such arrests, I have not seen a single Lazarus arise from the tomb of ventricular standstill, or "flatline"—no hearts restarted, no brains salvaged. They simply up and died.

I don't wish to put down CPR training. In rare instances—a near-drowning, a heart attack victim, a recent electrocution, a severe smoke inhalation—CPR and other resuscitation maneuvers save lives. But the ninety-year-old diabetic with end-stage heart failure? When that person's heart gives out, it's for keeps. That's one fact that TV dramas don't advertise: over 95 percent of resuscitations are unsuccessful. Of the few patients who are successfully revived, the majority die in a week.

What about all those near-death experiences? The shining light and all that? The heroism medals given for the quick-thinking Boy Scout with the CPR badge who saves the collapsed woman in the street? Unfortunately, many of these "resuscitations" are people who never had a cardiac arrest in the first place. When someone faints in hot weather, for example, the pulse temporarily slows so that even experienced paramedics can be fooled into thinking the heart has stopped cold. I once started chest compressions on a very obese woman who—or so I was told—had stopped breathing. She was so overweight that no one could feel a pulse anywhere in her body. I straddled her large abdomen with my legs and started heaving into her sternum with both hands. She awakened with a start and asked me exactly what I thought I was doing. Red-faced, I replied, "Would you believe saving your life?"

In the little spare time during the third year of medical school, I did a small research project in the immunology laboratory, studying how white cells migrated from tiny droplets of agarose. Agarose is a clear gelatin extracted from seaweed. A suspension of blood cells was mixed with warm agarose and deposited in little droplets onto a petri dish. The droplets, so small that their deposition required a low-power microscope, required great practice to get right.

Martha, a lab technician from England, taught me the delicate method of depositing the droplets. During the first few tries it became obvious that my hands trembled slightly under the microscope. Although I had no tremor to the unaided eye, the magnified image under the microscope revealed subtle finger gyrations which made it difficult to deposit a nicely rounded droplet. Martha's hands were rock steady, and she quickly grew impatient with me.

"Why are you so nervous, my dear?" she asked bluntly.

"I'm not nervous! Why should I be nervous about making silly little drops on a petri dish?" After all, I thought secretly, I have tormented people with nasogastric tubes!

"They are not silly," Martha snorted indignantly. "We're studying what causes multiple sclerosis and there isn't anything silly about that at all. No sir, not at all." Her British accent grew thicker when she was angry and

I sometimes enjoyed tormenting her just to hear her lapse into BBC speech.

"Well . . . I must have had too much coffee or something . . . that's all it is. We'll try again later."

She looked up from the microscope and peered at me skeptically with her green eyes. "All right, later then. You're not planning to be a brain surgeon with those hands are you, old man?"

This comment cut me to the bone, as if she could read my mind. I laughed nervously without making a reply.

When she had gone to another room, I played with the microsyringe, trying to steady my hands. After an hour of practice, I finally made a few decent droplets. It was the coffee, after all.

But Martha's parting words reverberated in my head. She didn't know what she was talking about! I could be anything in medicine I wanted to be. Even a brain surgeon! But how would I know that? There was only one way. I picked up the phone and called the neurosurgery office.

Yes, I would become "one of them."

4

A Night in the Street, a Night in the Chair

The clinical rotations of my final years of medical school passed quickly—except for psychiatry, which I found tedious. The patients were interesting, but the clinical pace was too slow for me. Assigned to the affective disorders unit, or ADU, I spent my six-week tour of duty in the university psychiatric institute. The ADU housed patients with severe disturbances of affect (psychiatry's term for mood). The ADU population consisted mostly of middle-aged women with major depression and young men with uncontrolled mania.

The ADU population harbored a fair number of schizophrenic patients as well. Schizophrenia isn't really a mood disorder—it's a thought disorder, or psychosis. But the institute had a limited number of beds on locked wards, and the ubiquitous schizophrenics were quartered in any empty beds.

Closet psychiatrists lurk everywhere, anxious to render armchair analyses of coworkers and friends. The workaholic in marketing, he's manic. Margaret next door sank into depression when her daughter went away to school. And John down the street—he's schizophrenic, totally bonkers. Amateurs toss these diagnoses about with no insight into their true manifestations. After encountering my first bona fide depressed, manic, and schizophrenic patients, the magnitude of their mood changes and aberrant behaviors shocked me.

Is that man in marketing manic simply because he's the first one into the office and the last out? How about a housing contractor I encountered who read the Bible, rode an exercise bike, dictated a letter to his secretary, and expounded on the dangers of having too many Jews in government—all at the same time?

Is the homemaker next door clinically depressed because she gets teary-eyed every morning looking at the photo of her daughter boarding a bus for college? How about a grandmother of three I saw, who spent eighteen hours a day sitting on her haunches, banging her head on the floor and repeating "God, kill me now" over and over again?

And the oddball down the street—is he schizophrenic because he wears black socks with white tennis shoes and talks to his tuberous begonias? How about a nurse's aide who plunged a bread knife into her vagina and partially cut away her own uterus because Satan told her that Julius Caesar's baby was in there?

Of all the illnesses I witnessed at the institute, the most fascinating was schizophrenia, a cruel and enigmatic disease which robs us of our most human quality: our reason. The word derives from the Greek for "split mind," and many still confuse schizophrenia with the very rare condition known as split, or multiple, personality disorder. Ironically, a schizophrenic barely possesses one complete personality, let alone two or more. Although many subclasses of the disorder exist, they all share common characteristics: apathy, deranged thought processes, the tendency to leap chaotically from topic to topic during a conversation (flight of ideas), feelings of persecution, and, finally, hallucinations—both auditory and visual (although the former are more common).

Schizophrenia stems from an imbalance in the brain chemical dopamine, the same chemical involved in the movement disorder Parkinson's disease. Prior to the introduction in 1952 of chlorpromazine, which normalizes the dopamine balance in schizophrenic brains, treatments of the disease ranged from the merely inane (dunking the patients in ice water) to the dangerous (lobotomy). Although a family of effective chlorpromazine-like drugs, known as antipsychotics, has been developed over the past forty years, the treatment of schizophrenia remains imperfect. Many patients become resistant to the medication, refuse to take it, or develop a Parkinson-like disability as a permanent side effect.

Some believe that schizophrenia is a modern illness, since ancient historians don't mention it. Others contend that earlier societies ignored schizophrenics—or treated them as possessed. How could such a dramatic syndrome be ignored, discounted into nonexistence?

Today, almost one in every hundred people in the United States is schizophrenic. One percent of the population suffers from the illness, yet its profile stays low and, on a dollars-per-new-case basis, schizophrenia* receives few government research funds. Given that they are virtually invisible now, the exclusion of schizophrenics from history becomes believeable.

Years ago, the great medical essayist Lewis Thomas wrote a poignant treatise on dead birds. He noted that

*See William T. Carpenter, Jr., and Robert W. Buchanan's excellent review article, "Schizophrenia," in *The New England Journal of Medicine* 330 (1994): 681–90.

we rarely see dead birds, certainly not in the numbers one would expect. The summer skies fill with live birds, pigeons choke our cities like rats with wings, gulls hover like bees around ships and beaches—yet their dead vanish. Aware of their impending demise, dying birds instinctively hide themselves away, perhaps to avoid contaminating the world of the living with their carrion. Schizophrenics do likewise. Like dead birds, their obscurity belies their swelled ranks. They seek haven on street grates, in halfway houses, in prisons, in attics.

The first schizophrenic I met face to face was Jake, a street dweller who wandered into the institute's evaluation center (a gentler title than "emergency room"). A winter evening had caused Jake to seek refuge from the cold . . . and "the wolves." The chief psychiatry resident instructed me and two other third-year medical students to chat with Jake in one of the interview areas. She handed us a three-inch-thick hospital folder marked "Jacob N. Guy." Jake was apparently a regular patron of the evaluation center.

The interview room was a cozy alcove with blue walls, soft chairs, and a long table of fake wood. Jake sat leaning his elbow on the table. He appeared to be about forty. Matted, filthy brown hair draped over his hunched shoulders, his tangled beard showed traces of gray. He wore a tattered spring jacket suited for April, not January. His face, white as Elmer's glue, had unremarkable features save for the eyes. Those wild eyes, unblinking black lasers, looked straight through me.

As we entered the room, my two colleagues pushed Jake's chart into my hand and then madly scrambled for the two chairs behind him, leaving me the sole chair facing him. My "friends" then waved their hands as a signal for me to proceed with the interview, as they smiled and held their noses. The room reeked of stale urine, an odor growing stronger as I leaned forward to introduce myself. I extended my hand to him, but Jake ignored me.

Thumbing quickly through the chart, I read that Jake had been a troubled child who had dropped out of school in the tenth grade. He drifted around Pennsylvania and Ohio, holding odd jobs until his behavior became too erratic even for menial work. A car wash in Steubenville fired him because he dried the same car a dozen times, fearing that the owner might die of germs unless he wiped them all away. A small landscaping company in Altoona could no longer deal with his bolting the lawnmower and cowering behind a tree for hours. A supermarket used him as a bag boy for less than a day.

Finally diagnosed as a schizophrenic at the age of twenty-five, Jake had been committed by the state to Woodville Mental Hospital, then released to a halfway house at the age of thirty-three. He spent less than a year there before taking to the streets, where he had lived ever since. He presented to the evaluation center every six months or so, when the weather outside got too formidable or when his most-feared hallucination, the wolves, haunted him. He would get a shot of Prolixin, an antipsychotic drug with effects lasting a month or more, and then be sent away. Rarely, he was admitted for a week or two.

I began timidly. "Jake, can you tell me why you are here to see us today?"

He said nothing for a few minutes as he sat and stared around the room, his mouth twisting and contorting—a side effect of the antipsychotic drugs. He then erupted with a single word:

"Wolves!"

"Wolves?"

"Yeah, shit, the wolves are out there, you know. They like us street meat. Christ, they chewed me up last year . . . If I had my gun, man, I could fight 'em . . . naw there're too many." He became more animated, his speech flowing in a rapid monotone. "They chased me down Grant Street last night and then they ate my buddy, Tommy. They go for the guts first, you know, flip you right over on your fuckin' back and start digging, like this"—Jake scraped frantically at the table with his nicotine-stained fingernails—"and then just pull your guts out and eat 'em. Shit and all. Poor Tommy, goddamn it . . . If I had my gun, he'd . . . but they don't let shitheads like me carry a gun anymore. Not since Nam. No sir—"

"You were in Vietnam?"

"I was in Vietnam, Russia, Cuba . . . the CIA sent me everywhere. Special Forces. Hamburger patties, that's all we are out there for them wolves. Yeah, Tommy and I were in Nam. That's when the wolves got wind of me. The Cong sent the wolves, and the bastards have been after me since 1971. Gook wolves, wolf gooks. Shit, let me in here so the gooks don't get me. Put me in a cage, I don't give a damn." The crazed look in his eyes faded into a sincere look of desperation and fear.

Jake's flight of ideas continued for another ten minutes, his thoughts ricocheting from subject to subject like a pinball. In Joseph Conrad's novel *Lord Jim*, Marlow observes that extracting truth from Jim was like trying to find out what was in a sealed metal box by beating upon it with a stick: you got a lot of noise, but no useful information. An excellent description of psychotic speech.

I broke off the interview and exited the room to seek out the psychiatry resident. We found her watching TV in the lounge.

"Well," she said upon seeing us, "what did you think of Jake?"

I related the story of the wolves and Tommy and Vietnam and the other observations I had hurriedly jotted down on his progress notes. "He's a little scary," I concluded.

"Schizophrenics are like rattlesnakes," she observed dryly. "They look scary, but they're far too frightened of *you* to be really dangerous. Personality disorders are a whole lot scarier, trust me. Tommy is Jake's brother, a system analyst for Coca-Cola. Jake talks about him, although they haven't spoken in years. Tommy was wounded in Vietnam while Jake was institutionalized. When Jake has an acute episode he usually says wolves are after him. Two years ago, it was a pack of dogs—the hallucination is being upgraded all the time. It's hard to tell if he really is afraid of his hallucinations or whether he just wants a night away from his cardboard box. I think it's the hallucinations—they can be frighteningly real to these people, like a waking nightmare. If he just wanted to be admitted for a few days, he could threaten violence or suicide and try to get a 302 that way—but he never has. Not yet, anyway." A 302 is an involuntary commitment to a psychiatric hospital, which can be imposed on patients only if they are perceived as an immediate physical threat to themselves or others.

The resident gave Jake his shot of Prolixin and returned him to the street. I watched him walk jerkily through the automated front doors, his gait bending under the weight of the brain-altering drugs, which had done little for him except make his movements as distorted as his thoughts. A wispy snow fell about him, dusting the walkways like confectioner's sugar. Jake pulled his spring jacket around his neck and wandered off into the blackness to face his wolves alone.

I graduated from medical school in May and began my surgical internship that July. Like medical school, internships consist of different rotations, providing the broadest possible experience before our careers funnel into single, narrow specialties. My first assignment as a full-fledged M.D. was cardiac surgery. The chest team at last!

Our cardiac service included both adults and children. A curious thing about illness: it strikes the very young and very old—but few in between. On the cardiac service, patients were either seventy years old and undergoing coronary artery bypass grafting (CABG, or "cabbages," as the residents affectionately called them), or three days old and undergoing a repair of a congenital FUH (fucked-up heart).

Interns did nothing of any consequence on the cardiac service. Not that we didn't work hard; there was a massive amount of inconsequential nothingness to do. To be stuck in the hospital for two or three days at a time was not unheard of. Every year, the police ticketed at least one cardiac intern for falling asleep at a red light while driving home.

Our purpose was to take night calls and to be human retractors in the operating room. During the day, I held quivering hearts upside down so that a vein graft could be sewn into their backsides. Immersed in iced saline during cardiopulmonary arrest, the hearts froze my fingers, and only hours after surgery did my frostbitten fingers regain their feeling.

The nights on call terrified me. Cardiac patients destabilize in an instant, and my knowledge of cardiac surgery bordered on the nonexistent. Opportunities for sleep were rare—the few moments between beeper pages were spent searching for drug dosages in the pocket-sized Washington Manual. We might be called to administer drugs to a 300-pounder one minute, and to medicate a four-pound infant the next.

I lived in constant fear of a patient "tamponade," when a blood clot forms around the post-op heart and smothers the life from it. If left untreated, even for a few minutes, tamponade kills swiftly. Faced with tamponade, we must tear out the skin sutures without delay; cut the bone wires to separate the halves of the freshly sawed sternum, or breastbone; and scoop the clot away from the heart. A set of suture-removal scissors and wire cutters sat taped at the bedside of every post-op cabbage for just such a delightful occasion.

Patients survived—provided the intern recognized the tamponade quickly and opened the chest immediately. There was no time for anesthetic during this emergency maneuver, however. Opening an awake patient's chest and showing them their own beating heart did not make my top-five list of favorite activities. When closing the chest cases on my call days, I prayed, "Please, dry this wound up, stop the bleeding . . . no tamponades tonight."

Heart surgery is a tough profession. A cardiac surgeon must complete six years of general surgery, followed by a two- or three-year cardiac fellowship. Operations stretched for hours; intraoperative deaths occurred frequently. Because of the hardships of training, cardiac programs attracted people with a Marine Corps attitude, residents so in love with their profession that the suffering became sweet nectar. They sported T-shirts that beamed: THE BEST WORK IN THE CHEST, and hung autographed pictures of Michael DeBakey in their lockers.

My chief cardiac fellow, Maggie, exemplified the drill-sergeant demeanor. The ER called Maggie and me one night to evaluate an elderly woman flown in from another hospital. The woman was barely clinging to life. A ventilator tethered her to earth, else she would have expired hours earlier. A cardiac catheterization, done at the first hospital, had disclosed a blown mitral valve. The mitral valve, stopcock between left atrium and left ventricle, had stuck in the open position, its mechanism damaged by a fresh heart attack. With each beat, blood drove backward into the atrium, not forward into her body. Unless replaced with a synthetic valve, the broken mitral would kill her before the sun rose.

Maggie, fresh from two straight cabbage procedures, was clearly tired. She scanned the cath report with a heavy-lidded stare, then shook her head slowly. I expected her to pound her fist with rage, angry at the unceasing workload. I had seen residents in other fields crumble under the onslaught of a never-ending day. Instead, she looked at me with a wicked grin. "Frank, we've got a mitral valve to do! Oh, baby, this is great . . . YOU GOTTA LOVE THIS!!" She gleefully pranced to a phone to call the OR. She should take up bowling, I thought, just for a change of pace.

In the uterus, the fetus breathes through the umbilical-cord blood, not the lungs. The unborn possess an elaborate bypass system which shunts blood away from their water-logged lungs and into the mother's placenta. At the moment of birth, this bypass system shuts down, clotting off the umbilical cord and diverting blood to the virgin lungs.

The *in utero* blood shunt carries two consequences for the cardiac surgeon: The closure of the shunt at birth occasionally fails and must be completed with a knife; and, since the normal circulation of blood is superfluous until after birth, some truly terrible heart malformations pass undetected until the delivery room, requiring the surgeon to rebuild the heart from scratch.

Although many malformations have been described and named—tetralogy of Fallot, total anomalous venous return, hypoplastic left ventricle—malformations are as individual as fingerprints, hence the less restrictive "fucked-up heart" category.

Some malformations kill the infant minutes after birth; others are mild, and their correction can be deferred for years. Most deformities, however, fall between these two extremes, producing a heart good enough to sustain life for a month or two but not good enough to last years. In these instances, the surgeon must decide whether the defect is correctable. If not, the child is left to die, or referred to the heart-transplantation waiting list.

Baby girl McKenna had entered the world with a small right ventricle. This pumping chamber receives depleted venous blood from the body and flushes it into the lungs, where it is replenished with oxygen. A month premature, she had arrived before her parents could agree upon a name. Her condition had deteriorated rapidly after birth, and she was sent to our pediatric heart service during one of my nights off. When I arrived in the pediatric ICU to make rounds at 5 A.M., little B.G. McKenna, a blue blob on maximal life support, awaited the next operating-room slot. Maggie sat in her surgical scrubs and rocked slowly in a large wooden rocking chair—known as *the* chair by cardiac interns.

"I don't know what we can do for this munchkin," she said, sipping from a vending machine cup. "Hartley and I are doing her as soon as they finish the trauma patient that's in the heart room." Hartley was the chief of pediatric cardiac surgery.

That's great, I thought. I was on call for the night. B.G. and I were sure to have a fun time together. Babies this small can't tolerate the heart-lung machine, and are done instead under "profound hypothermia." The infant is packed in ice until suspended animation occurs, and the heart is stopped and repaired as quickly as possible.

Certain species of frogs and fish can be frozen solid and rethawed with no apparent injury. But babies are neither frog nor fish. Without the protein antifreezes that circulate in those animals, they emerge from profound hypothermia near death, their blood-clotting mechanisms deranged, their livers reeling, their brains dysfunctional. I looked at *the* chair, now occupied by Maggie—the command seat for the pediatric heart patients in the children's ICU. We spent many nights in it, wrapped in an afghan and rocking nervously, watching patients too unstable to be unattended.

B.G.'s surgery commenced later that morning and finished around five o'clock. Having scrubbed on cabbages until about eight, I finally wandered down to the pediatric ICU for signout at nine. Maggie awaited me, anxious to sign out B.G. before leaving. The service was quiet . . . except for B.G. As I expected, the problem for the night.

Surgical soap stained her scrawny little body orange from her neck to feet. Heating lamps dangled above the bed, to restore warmth to her frigid body. She looked like a little cornish hen roasting under the heat lamps of a delicatessen.

Maggie handed me an index card. "Here, I've calculated the doses of the resuscitation drugs for her weight. I think everything is there—epi, bicarb, bretylium . . . The nurses know the defib settings, they'll help you with that. You've taken infant CPR? Good. You'll need it. She's going to have a rough night, but if she makes it twelve or twenty-four hours, she has a shot. The parents have just left. . . . We're all counting on you. I want her alive tomorrow morning. You know how to reach me if you get up to your ass in alligators. . . . So long."

Maggie left. I dragged the heavy rocking chair beside the rotisserie bed and plopped myself in for the night. Gazing at the monitor, I watched the little squiggles that B.G.'s damaged heart traced across the fluorescent screen. So far, so good.

I dozed for a short time. A nurse shook me awake. "Her pressure's falling," she whispered.

I cleared the cobwebs from my head and ordered an infusion of albumin and an increase in her dopamine, an intravenous drug which stimulates the failing heart muscle. (The drug dopamine is the same as the brain chemical dopamine which is deranged in schizophrenics. The human body uses many chemicals in multiple roles.) B.G. stabilized for an hour before her blood pressure dipped precipitously again. Despite more albumin, the pressure bottomed out completely and her heart fibrillated wildly.

I jumped from the chair and started cardiac compressions on her tiny chest with my index and middle fingers. I ordered a bolus of epinephrine (also know as adrenaline) and the fibrillation reverted to a normal rhythm. The blood pressure went up to ninety. Breathing a sigh of relief, I went to the nurses' station and called Maggie at home, informing her of the successful resuscitation.

"What do you want, a medal?" she croaked. "What is it, two A.M.? You got hours to go before she's stable . . . and go easy on the epi; her perfusion is poor as it is and I don't want her fingers to die. Push the fluid harder."

My ego deflated, I went back to the chair. Maggie was right about the epinephrine. B.G.'s fingertips grew more discolored by the hour. Like Mephistopheles, epinephrine will do your bidding—for a price. The increase in blood pressure and heart contractility after an epi infusion comes at the expense of blood flow to the limbs. Too much epi and the hands and feet will become gangrenous.

Another hour passed before the hypotension and fibrillation returned. More CPR, more albumin. Some lidocaine and bretylium. A blast from the miniature defibrillator. Nothing worked. I gave yet another bolus of epi. Again, the pressure shot up, the heart rhythm stabilized. B.G.'s fingers and toes became darker and more mottled.

To prevent another round of hypotension, I increased the intravenous infusions drastically, but her lungs filled with fluid and the oxygen level in her arteries fell dramatically. To counteract this, I gave her Lasix, a strong diuretic. The Lasix had no effect. The urine output slowed, no doubt due to lack of blood flow to the kidneys: another side effect of the epi.

The fibrillation came again.

They are all counting on me. The words rang in my tired brain. Her mom and dad, Hartley, Maggie . . . they are counting on me to keep this baby alive. I ordered another bolus of epinephrine. Take this child's fingers, Satan. Faustus selling his soul for another hour of stability, another hour of fitful sleep in the chair. . . .

The epi kept the devil's bargain: the blood pressure soared and a sinus rhythm once more hammered its way across the monitor screen. I glanced at the clock: four-thirty. Time for rounds soon. My eyes closed.

Maggie grabbed my arm. Disoriented, I jumped from the chair and to B.G.'s bed. Empty. The heat lamps dark. Looking again at the clock, I realized that I had been asleep for over two hours! Panic overcame me. What had I slept through? They had been counting on me.

Maggie chuckled at my frenzy. "Relax."

"Where's the baby? Did she go back to the OR?"

"No, I shut off her ventilator an hour ago. She's in the morgue. Actually, her parents wanted her shut off last night before I left, but I forgot."

"In the morgue? You forgot what? What do you mean, they wanted her shut off last night?" I was confused, furious.

"Hartley met with them after surgery. You see, we couldn't repair the right ventricle. All we could do was enlarge it with a Teflon patch, but Teflon doesn't pump blood, you know. We knew she was a goner when she left the table. The family was very reasonable—the mother's an ER nurse across town—they couldn't see prolonging things and they gave us the okay to halt support. I just figured we could wait until morning to do the deed."

"Why didn't you tell me all this last night? Why did you let me sit in this fucking chair all night thinking I was making some baby's fingers drop off?"

Maggie's smirk vanished. "Your night wasn't such a waste, was it? You learned how to resuscitate a baby, how to face crisis, what drugs to use and what problems they can cause. I bet you won't forget the doses of those drugs for a while, either. They are burned into your brain. You did a good job. Not many people can keep a Teflon heart beating for ten hours. Now I know I can count on you to handle a baby with a real chance of living."

"You could have told me that she was a goner—I was crapping in my drawers."

"No. Then you wouldn't have been under the gun. Pressure's part of the deal. Anybody can sing in the shower, but how many can sing in front of an audience, huh? Pressure makes all the difference in the world."

5

The Museum of Pain

> Pleasure is oft a visitant; but pain clings cruelly to us.
> —John Keats

Pain is the price we pay for mobility. Since the dawn of life creatures have segregated into two camps: motionless food-makers and migrating food foragers. Creatures in the first camp learned to draw energy from their immediate environments. Plants turn chloroplasts to the sun and use photosynthesis to manufacture glucose, while deep-sea creatures harness heat arising from thermal vents on the ocean floor.

Creatures in the second camp sprouted tails, legs, fins, and wings and set off to eat the food makers, or each other. Lacking a clever trick like photosynthesis, the food foragers came up with a new invention: the nervous system. To say that the nervous system evolved so that animals could sense and respond to their surroundings is only partly correct. Anything alive, brainy or not, must be able to sense and respond to its surroundings. Bacteria "know" when the ambient moisture is too low, and form into spores which are more resistant to drying. A tree senses when autumn comes and jettisons its leaves as the sunlight fades.

But these responses are relatively simple and slow, taking hours, days, even weeks to complete. Moreover, no-brain creatures such as trees and bacteria have only tiny repertoires of stereotyped responses. The tree adapts to the seasons but, having no place to run, falls victim to sudden, life-threatening events—forest fire, bark-eating deer, beavers' incisors. As compensation for this help-lessness, nature blessed the mindless tree with ignorant bliss. The oak feels no pain from the lumberjack's saw. The pine does not cry out in agony as lightning bursts its trunk asunder.

Animals, constantly at odds with a changing environ-ment or with other animals, could not survive with the tree's small number of adaptive mechanisms. Peripatetic organisms need complex responses which can be cus-tomized in milliseconds—they need a nervous system. Although sensation and adaptation can occur in the absence of brain tissue, these skills are elevated to a new level of speed and diversity by an organ system devoted solely to cognition. The primordial ganglion protobrains became the digital computers of biology, leaving the abacus-like reasoning of the plant kingdom in the dust.

As always, there was a terrible price to pay for this new technology. Animals dependent for survival upon the complex software of nerve cells and the delicate clockwork of churning limbs are very vulnerable to injury. Yes, the big stupid tree doesn't know enough to run away from fire—but it can lose over half its branches and live. A squirrel with one broken leg is as good as dead. In the natural world, where any breach of the skin can mean infection and death, an animal must stay out of harm's way. Like the earliest computers, the earliest brains were pretty dim. The only way to keep animals equipped with "first generation" brain hardware out of trouble was through aversion: dangerous things became painful things. Pain became the taskmaster of the animal world.

Unfortunately, the blossoming of our magnificent forebrains did not free us from the bondage of animal pain. We are now smart enough to learn abstractly that fire hurts without having to experience it firsthand, yet we still endure the agony of burns. The pain pathways that torment us with toothaches, menstrual cramps, and bee stings have progressed little from the days of the walnut-brained stegosaurus writhing in a predator's jaws. The continuing need for pain in humans no doubt derives from the stupidity of young children, who, as any parent can attest, feel compelled to seek what does and does not hurt for themselves.

The pain pathways have no "off" switch. Pain lingers long after its biological usefulness has passed. Although a pain alerting us to the presence of curable cancer is a valuable torment, cancer pain doesn't have the merciful sense to cease after the cancer has spread to a terminal stage. The nervous system *does* possess two means of limiting pain perception: chemicals known as endorphins and a spinal-cord switching mechanism called "gating." They are far from perfect in their natural state but can be augmented with the help of medical technology.

Endorphins, natural substances related to morphine, are released in times of stress. Like morphine they are very good for acute, severe pain, but not so effective for mild or chronic pain. Endorphins evolved so that wounded animals could function, at least for a short while. Example: a doe, mortally wounded by a car, ignores the pain and crawls away in search of her fawn.

Endorphins permit a running back to keep chugging for the goal line oblivious to the fact that his arm was broken on the line of scrimmage.

Endorphins also perform a true mercy service, anesthetizing an animal trapped by a carnivore. Those people who have survived being caught in the jaws of lions or grizzly bears speak of the warm, insensate calm that flowed through them as they succumbed to being eaten alive.

The gating phenomenon is a second mechanism for blunting painful sensations. The spinal cord is like a collection of railway tracks: sensations ascend within it like freight trains running on those tracks. Each sensory modality (pain, temperature, fine touch, heavy pressure) is like freight carried to the brain on separate trains. Access to the brain is limited, however. Only so many trains enter at once, only so much freight is unloaded into our consciousness. When one sensation is dominant, the others are blocked, "gated."

The gating mechanism occurs with the other senses as well. If, as we are listening to one conversation at a cocktail party, we are then engaged in another, the voices in the original conversation fade into the background. Likewise, we find it difficult to smell two strong odors at once. Many commercial products operate on the gating principle. Bathroom deodorizers don't remove foul odors; they gate them from our brains by superimposing a stronger, more pleasant odor. Noise "masking" devices for airplane travelers gate out the annoying whine of an airplane engine with a more soothing white noise.

Pain can be gated from the brain by superimposing another sensation. If we scald a hand with hot water, we immediately rub the burned area. We are inately seeking to gate the pain out, to prevent the pain train from pulling into the brain station. Pain gating is the mechanism behind the old coaching aphorism "Walk it off." Migraine sufferers knead their temples; sufferers of leg cramps knead their calves. Gating underlies the effectiveness of massage, ice packs, heating pads, liniments, and acupuncture. Attempts to gate pain can be taken to perverse extremes. Napoleon, troubled in his later years by kidney stones, routinely burned himself with a candle to divert his attention from abdominal pain.

Neurosurgeons deal in pain on a daily basis. Pain in the head, pain in the face, pain in the arms, pain in the legs, pain in the neck, pain in the back—all, essentially, a pain in the ass for patient and doctor alike. Over two-thirds of all neurosurgical operations are for pain control—or, more properly, the alleviation of suffering.

There is a profound difference between pain and suffering. All animals feel pain. Only humans suffer. Pain is a physical sensation; suffering is an emotional state induced by pain. Suffering is pain coupled with uncertainty, depression, frustration, anger, fear, despair. We can have intense pain but not suffer. A stubbed toe, a shin whacked against a coffee table, a softball to the groin, a paper cut, a mouth ulcer—all may elicit extreme pain with little suffering. We know these pains are temporary. We know that they will go away and that they bode no long-term ill for our bodies.

But what of a woman who thinks she is cured of her breast cancer and then develops a minor backache? Her mind is troubled. Is it the cancer again? Until she finds out, she will suffer greatly. That small backache will become like a nail driven into her spine until she knows what it signifies. When told that all the tests are negative for cancer, she feels better instantly. No pain medications could accomplish this. The pain is the same, but the suffering is eased. In a sense, suffering is pain augmented by a bleak imagination. We construct dismal scenarios for our unexplained miseries: That toothache must mean a root canal; that hand stiffness is rheumatoid arthritis; that heartburn could be coronary artery disease.

Hippocrates once said that the chief function of medicine is to entertain patients until they heal themselves. On the pain service, we didn't entertain our patients; far from it. We took their pain away as best we could.

Of course, sometimes we had to poke holes in their heads to do it.

The very first morning of my residency, Gary and Eric took me to the neurosurgery floor and introduced me to some of the pain patients on the service. I had little previous experience with the pain service. At the time of my medical student rotation, there were relatively few pain service patients in the hospital. I had avoided even that handful, concentrating instead on the more "interesting" cases like brain abscesses, pituitary tumors, and carotid aneurysms. A medical student can get away with ignoring tedious problems in favor of more challenging ones. But residency was different. Medical school is five parts learning to one part servitude; the ratio is reversed in residency.

We halted at room nine, a private room.

"Room nine," Eric whispered, "Mr. van Buren. Status post-five laminectomies for ruptured lumbar discs. He's from Boston, runs an investment company or something. He has chronic right leg pain and has been on oral morphine for the last six months. We put in an epidural spinal cord stimulator yesterday and externalized it. The guy's now playing with it to see if any of the settings make his pain go away. If not, we yank it. If it does, we internalize it to an antenna and send him to a detox unit."

Gary explained that the spinal stimulator's gate mechanism permits pain to be masked by a simultaneous sensation, such as touching or rubbing. Not surprisingly, people with chronic sciatica find it impractical to go around rubbing their legs all day. To exploit the gate mechanism, devices which continuously stimulate the touch nerves have been marketed. The simplest is the transepidermal nerve stimulator, or TENS unit, which consists of surface electrodes taped to the skin and hooked to a portable battery supply. The TENS unit provides a gentle "buzz" to the affected skin, akin to the low-level shock felt when touching the transformer of a toy electric train set. In patients with "failed back syndrome," or FBS, severe leg pain from a damaged spinal nerve lingers even after one or more "successful" operations to remove a ruptured back disc. Many FBS sufferers can get by with a TENS unit attached to their affected leg all day.

Eventually the TENS unit fails, though, and more masking stimulation is needed. To accomplish this, a thin electrode is threaded under the skin, between the vertebrae and directly over the spinal cord, into an area known as the spinal epidural space (the same area anesthetized during labor and delivery). The electrode is initially brought out through the skin and hooked to a compact control box to allow the patient to experiment with different spinal stimulation settings. If the patient gets relief, he or she is returned to the OR and the electrode is put under the skin and connected to a subcutaneous antenna. The stimulator is then completely internalized and safe from infection. Stimulating signals are broadcast to the spinal cord electrode via a radio transmitter hooked to the belt or worn over the shoulder like a purse.

We entered the room. Mr. van Buren, dressed in expensive-looking pajamas, sat in a chair by his bed. He was a large man with a pleasant, ruddy face and coarse black hair cropped short, almost in a crew cut. On his lap lay a small beige box, the size of a pack of cigarettes, with several buttons and dials on one side. Two thin wires sprouted from the top of the box and disappeared into the front of his pajama top. He looked to be deep in concentration as his thick fingers twiddled the knobs on the box.

"Good morning, Mr. van Buren. Have you had any luck?" asked Gary in his best professional tone.

"I can get it to buzz a little around my butt cheeks when I use the square wave pulse and turn the frequency to . . . here."

"Does that help?"

"A little, but it feels like my pants are warm, like I'm pissing myself all the time. I'm not sure that's any better than the pain."

"Mr. van Buren, this is Dr. Vertosick," Eric spoke, "and he's joining our team for the next six months. You'll be seeing him every morning now."

The man looked up from his box and smiled politely.

"Nice to meet you, Doctor."

"I understand you have had five disc surgeries?"

"Yes . . . the first was in 1974 . . . but here, let me show you."

The man reached over to his nightstand, opened the top drawer, and produced a leather-bound folder with the

words "Myelograms and records of A. van Buren" sten-
ciled on the front cover in gold leaf. "Have a seat, Dr.
Ferblowstick."

He proceeded to explain the saga of his many operations in great detail, turning the pages with the slow
intensity of a newlywed showing off a wedding album.
"Look, here was right after the second operation . . . there
was a little scarring around the fifth lumbar root, but no
arachnoiditis yet. . . . My surgeon thought that this might
be a disc fragment here, and he looked again in 1981. . . .
Here the arachnoiditis got bad . . ."

Among the photos of myelograms and CT scans
and operative notes were other memorabilia: labels from
bottles of narcotics, letters containing second surgical
opinions, insurance forms, articles on holistic healing
and the power of positive thinking. He grew more excited
as he spoke, spouting his tale of vertebral vivisection at
the hands of three surgeons with as much glee as a fisherman recounting his battle with a prize marlin. He didn't
seem to be in any pain at all.

"Mr. van Buren," Gary interrupted him, "tell Dr. *Vertosick* what your pain is like now."

"Oh," he replied, still grinning, "it's awful, excruciating. It's like an army of red-hot earthworms crawling
up inside my leg, wriggling and writhing day in and day
out. Occasionally, I get a groin pain, over here, that's like
a C-clamp being slowly twisted down on my pubic
bone."

"Thanks, we'll see you this afternoon . . . try turning
the amplitude down and the frequency up. If that doesn't
work, we may have to take you back to the OR and
repositon the electrode."

We exited the room and walked a little way down

the hall. When we were far enough away from room nine, Gary spoke: "Well, class, what did Mr. van Buren teach us?"

"Ah, that the electrode . . ."

"Forget the friggin' electrode. Is this guy in pain?"

I was confused.

"Is he in pain?"

"I guess so?"

Gary motioned me over to another room, room eighteen. Lying in the bed was a pale, wasted man. "Hey, Mr. Angelo, it's Gary. Tell young Dr. Vertosick what your leg pain is like."

"I dunno." The man's voice was thin, weak. "It hurts like hell is all I can say. Right about here. Real sore."

"Thanks, Mr. Angelo." We darted back into the hallway again.

"Mr. Angelo has a malignant sarcoma eating into his lower back and right lumbar plexus," Gary continued, "and he's in agony. Does he say he has goddamned electric earthworms in his leg or some such shit like that? No. He says 'I'm real sore.' He also uses about one-tenth the morphine that room nine uses. Why? Because he has legitimate pain and he isn't nuts. Another rule of thumb: The more bizarre the description of the pain, the more likely it is to be a psychiatric delusion. Phrases like 'I have little gnomes with branding irons running all over my face' or 'The hooves of a thousand angry horses are thundering in my head' should immediately make you suspicious that something else is going on. People with real pain don't say 'excruciating.' The word 'excruciating' literally means to feel the pain of crucifixion. Since hardly anybody knows what it's like to be crucified anymore, no one is entitled to use that word, in my humble opinion."

"Look at that guy!" Eric chimed in. "My kid's pictures don't get as much attention as his X rays! He's *becoming* his pain. It's part of his identity. He'll be in pain until it's time for him to make the horizontal call from a brass-handled phone booth—which won't be long if he keeps slurping up oral morphine."

We proceeded down the hallway to room eleven.

"Room eleven," said Eric. "Mrs. Rubinstein, atypical face pain. Had a microvascular decompression of the fifth cranial nerve three days ago. Still has face pain, same as pre-op. Wound looks good, no headache—thank God for small favors. . . . Husband Ben by her side, as usual." A microvascular decompression is the act of padding arteries away from the cranial nerves at the base of the brain using small Teflon sponges; it was the first operation I had seen—or at least started to see until Gary plunged the drill into the patient's cerebellum and made me flee the OR.

The body has twelve pairs of cranial nerves, so named because they exit from the brain itself, not from the spinal cord. The cranial nerves mediate the sensory and motor functions of the head and neck. The first cranial nerves are the olfactory nerves, which convey the sense of smell; the second cranial nerves the optic nerves, which convey the sense of sight; and so on. The fifth cranial nerve conveys sensations from the face. It is also called the trigeminal nerve, from the Greek phrase meaning "three origins," because the main nerve branches into three divisions: V1 (called vee-one, even though the "V" is meant to be the Roman numeral five, not the letter), which supplies sensation to the forehead and eyes; V2, which supplies the cheeks, upper teeth, and upper lip; and V3, which supplies the jaw, lower teeth, and lower lip. The trigeminal nerve is somewhat rudimentary in humans compared to the nerves of lower animals, such as mice or cats, which have whiskers and depend upon keen facial sensation for their survival.

"*Atypical* facial pain?" I asked. "Is that like trigeminal neuralgia?"

"No." Gary answered sharply. "It isn't anything like trigeminal neuralgia, or tic. People with tic have stabbing pains in one, or perhaps two, divisions of the nerve. The pains are elicited by sensations in the affected area: brushing the teeth, cold air or water hitting the face, chewing. Atypical patients have pain all the time, describing it as burning or aching and not shocklike."

"Does surgery help this?"

"Judge for yourself."

Mrs. Rubinstein, an attractive woman of about forty, wore a sexy nightgown and large, dangling gold earrings. The right earring smacked repeatedly against the shaven, sutured wound behind her ear as she turned her head to greet us. A bald man sat in a chair beside her bed.

"Mr. and Mrs. Rubinstein, this is Dr. Vertosick. As of today, he's a brain surgeon. How's your face?"

"Awful, just ahhhwful." She had a heavy New York accent—I wasn't versed enough to tell exactly what part of the city it was from. "What can I say, it's worse than it was before, I'm telling you. Like grease from a doughnut frier being poured onto my face all of the time. My God, I thought that this was really going to do it for me. Right, Benjamin?" (A vigorous nod from the bald man.) "The people at the Mayo Clinic and Hopkins told me that *this* was the place to go, but I don't know. Doughnut grease,

I'm telling you, doughnut grease. One Percocet just isn't holding me. I told you people that I need two every four hours or I'm not fit to live with. When we were at Cornell, they tried to switch me to Motrin, but what a scene I made!"

"Is it still hurting you . . . all the way to here?" Eric reached over and gently touched the woman's hairline at the top of her forehead. She winced.

"Yeah, yeah."

"But not here." Eric drubbed his index finger in her scalp, just behind the hairline.

"No, not the scalp . . . just the face hurts. Doughnut grease, scalding doughnut grease. My God, I swear one day I'll wake up and big strips of scalded skin will peel off on my pillow!"

"Is your pain excruciating?" I asked.

"Definitely."

Gary's face became stern. "Well, we'll see what the boss has to say. Good thing the mister's here to take care of you, huh?"

"Yeah, he's such a dear."

"So long."

"Doctor?"

"Yes, Mrs. Rubinstein?"

"My Percocet?"

"I'll have to check with your attending surgeon first; I'm sorry."

Back into the hallway, Gary started grilling me again.

"Anything funny about her pain?"

"She uses that graphic imagery you were talking about with Mr. van Buren."

"Uh-huh. But what about the distribution of her pain?"

"It stops at the hairline and doesn't go into her scalp?"

"Bingo! And where does the distribution of the trigeminal nerve stop?"

"At the vertex of the head, almost back to the occipital area."

"Bingo again! Society defines the face as being from the hairline down, while the brain considers almost the whole head as the face. Patients with V1 tic have pain extending well into their scalps. I've seen patients who haven't washed or combed their hair on the affected side of their heads for days or weeks because they can't touch their scalps. Her pain distribution follows a culturally defined area, not an anatomically defined one. Her pain has to be psychiatric in origin."

"But we did a craniotomy on her," I observed.

"There is no way to be sure she doesn't have some component of tic pain," said Eric. "On the pain service, we have to assume all pain to be real, organic, and that the pain makes people eccentric, not vice versa. In any pain patient, no matter how bizarre the history, may be a kernel of real pain, like a splinter at the bottom of a festering sore."

"So the pain service doesn't refuse anybody?"

"No," answered Gary, "and room twenty-two is a case in point."

In room twenty-two was a wispy little man in his mid-twenties. He was thin to the point of pathological anorexia, his face covered with blemishes and his hair thinning in random spots. An odd collection of items lined the man's windowsill, each with a note card taped upon it. Across the top of the window was a large banner that read "Harry Gottlieb's Museum of Pain."

After I was introduced, Harry, who had suffered from chronic headaches for years, showed me his museum.

"This is the Dodgers cap which used to take away my pain whenever I wore it. It quit working for some reason. And this . . . this is the TENS unit they gave me at the pain clinic in Erie. It really didn't help much at all. I even shaved my head so that the electrode patches would stick better, but that didn't make any difference. And the patches cost a lot of money, so I quit using it. . . . These are a collection of the pain medications I've tried over the past eight years . . ."

I rummaged through the bottles: Dilaudid, Percocet, Elavil, all the bottles large—and empty.

"Mr. Gottlieb, what's your headache like?" I asked.

"Like a big railroad spike that some large man is hammering right into the top of my head. And it's one of those square spikes, not sharp at all. Dull. Pounding right down into the center of my head, right here."

One of the staff surgeons had recently placed a midbrain stimulator into Mr. Gottlieb. This device is a higher-powered version of the epidural stimulator inserted at the very top of the pain pathways.

"Did your operation help you?" I pointed to the incision on his balding scalp.

"Yes, oh, my yes. The spike feels sharp now, not dull and square anymore."

I thanked him for the tour of his "museum" and we went back to our rounds. We left him scurrying about his windowsill, tidying up his Museum of Pain for the next visitors.

I stopped and confronted Gary and Eric before continuing with rounds. "You guys are pulling my leg, right? These can't be typical patients—the only patient with real pain was that Italian man with the sarcoma."

Gary stopped me. "Let's be serious. These people have

real problems and we shouldn't make light of them. And we can't be sure whether they are having pain or not. If someone ever invents an accurate pain-o-meter, then that person should get a Nobel Prize. But for now, the only way we judge pain is by what the patient says. These people are feeling some kind of pain, if only psychic pain. They need help; I'm just not sure if they need *our* help. But there is no way to know for sure, so we give them the benefit of the doubt. If we fail, we send them to the pain clinic, where the anesthesiologists, psychiatrists, and social workers take over."

We finished rounds. My mind was troubled. When I first started working in our local steel mill, I thought I'd be making steel, but I'd spent all of my time shoveling grease. I'd entered neurosurgery to help people, but these people seemed beyond help. My mother had once suggested that I not go to medical school, that I stay in the factory, since that was as good a job as any. Was she right?

The pain patients made up only half of the service. The other half consisted of ER consults, trauma victims, and the elective patients of the other university neurosurgeons. We were also responsible for the in-house neurosurgical consults, which were sometimes interesting, sometimes tedious.

The university's medical center had a diverse patient population, bringing problems ranging from spinal pain in a melanoma patient to brain mass in a liver transplant recipient. The most common consults were for mundane complaints—say, benign backaches, or requests for the neurosurgery resident on call to perform a lumbar puncture, or LP. Because neurosurgeons violate the brain's natural barriers to infection, any post-operative fever in one of our patients may herald a bacterial meningitis. Fever in a post-op head case mandated a lumbar puncture, known to laymen as a "spinal tap," so that some of the cerebrospinal fluid, or CSF, could be sent for a white cell count, glucose measurement, and bacteriological cultures. When we were busy, I would do ten to twelve LPs a day. Medical residents, in comparison, might do ten or twelve a year, while other specialties may do less than that in a career. By virtue of our experience and availability, we were the LP mavens of the health center.

The procedure consists of turning a patient on his or her side, numbing a small patch of skin in the middle of the lower back, and plunging a six-inch-long needle into the spinal canal. (It's best not to show the needle to the patient, I have discovered.) The fluid is left to drip into sterile plastic containers, like maple sap from a tree.

In younger patients, a spinal tap can be trivially easy. Not so in the aged. As we grow older, the small openings in our spines—tiny windows between the vertebral laminae which permit the entrance of the LP needle—are slowly occluded by the advancing bone spurs of degenerative arthritis. This makes LP's very difficult affairs in elderly patients, sometimes requiring many minutes of blind probing with the needle before a portal into the spine can be located. One patient suggested that a divining rod might be useful, to point the way to watery paydirt.

More often than not, the failed LP was a result of inexperience, of a medical student or an intern's sticking the needle far off the mark. Patients will tolerate only so much amateur prospecting in their bones and nerves before they order the procedure abandoned. But if meningitis is suspected, there is no waiting for tomorrow: the test must be done immediately. When the medical interns cannot obtain a successful LP, neurosurgery is called to save the day. This was not a pleasant assignment. We frequently had to try again in a hornet-mad patient whose back looked like a sprinkler head. Ah, but the sweet pleasure of passing the needle effortlessly into a ravaged spine in seconds, when other doctors had tried for an hour or more! All I needed was a ten-gallon hat and I was off into the sunset. Shucks, ma'am, 'twern't nothin'!

This dire need to obtain spinal fluid in a case of suspected meningitis illustrates how the physician's job, particularly a surgeon's, differs from most others. In medicine, results count, not effort. *Get spinal fluid.* That's all, just get it. And soon. Nobody cares how tired you are, or how much the patient bitched, or how the hospital didn't have a long enough spinal needle, or that the patient was a thousand years old or weighed a thousand pounds. Nobody cares that your technique was correct. Just get spinal fluid. Use fluoroscopy. Sit the patient up. Stand him on his head. Give him Valium. Do what it takes; just do it. His life may well depend upon success.

My last physics course as an undergraduate was Mathematical Methods in Physics. On the first day of class, the professor informed us that there would be only one test, the final exam, and that it would consist of only one problem. He wanted only the answer to that problem, accurate to four decimal places, written on a scrap of paper above our name. If we were correct to all four decimal places, we'd get an A. If not, we'd fail. Simple. There were immediate howls of protest from myself and others. One test? One answer? Didn't he even want to know how we set up the problem? If we even knew what we were doing?

"No," he replied. "Welcome to the real world, where people only want answers—correct, accurate answers. If a bridge collapses and kills forty people, who do you think cares whether the engineers set up the problem correctly? In life, there is no partial credit for being half right. If you want to accomplish anything important, you have to be totally right—and be willing to take the consequences if you are not."

As the professor argued, all real-world occupations require a certain level of performance. The physician's performance must be perfect, however, and it must be perfect right now. In a lifetime, a surgeon performs thousands of operations and makes hundreds of thousands of decisions regarding medications, antibiotics, when to operate, when not to operate. Complicating matters is the fact that these decisions often must be made quickly and with incomplete information. Call a lawyer at three in the morning and ask to have a coherent defense strategy laid out right now! Wake an airline pilot from a dead sleep and expect him to pull the plane out of a nose dive right now! Take a car to a mechanic and say fix it right now— not a day from now, or an hour from now.

One night I was summoned for an emergency LP on a young man from the medical service, admitted that day in a stuporous condition and now nearly comatose. His brain CT showed nothing unusual. He had a slight fever and a stiff neck, and the diagnosis of bacterial meningitis had to be ruled out. Both the intern and the resident on the house medical service had tried to get spinal fluid and had no luck. They called for the radiologist to do the procedure under fluoroscopy, but she refused to come in from home until I had given it my best shot. She paged me to ask if I could spare her a night trip to the hospital, as her daughter wasn't feeling well.

There was the usual bedside scene: a naked man on his side in a fetal pose, his back purple from failed LP attempts, brown prep solution staining the sheets and floor. A dozen blood-soaked gauze sponges littered the bed, the wreckage of a prepackaged LP tray strewn across the patient's nightstand.

The man was very tan, even in places that shouldn't *be* tan, and he had short, bleached-blond hair. Gold chains adorned his neck and right ankle. He had an excellent physique.

"Is he awake?" I asked. "Any sign of trauma?"

"He moans; that's about it," replied the medical intern, still wearing her bloodstained latex gloves. "And no, no sign of trauma."

"He sure looks healthy for a sick guy ... What's the name?"

"Roger Doe."

"Roger Doe? Any relation to John?"

"Everybody who comes to the ER without ID is called Doe. They rotate first names to keep the record room from being clogged with John Does. We're up to the *R*'s already."

"No kidding! Like naming hurricanes. What's wrong with him?" I asked as I pulled on gloves and began to probe the mauled back in search of a virgin interspace. I immediately detected the error of the intern's failed attempts: she was far too low and had been skewering the hard sacrum, or tailbone. Nothing but blood there.

"He came in like this, found unresponsive on the street and brought in by the police from downtown," the intern continued. "He was probably robbed after he collapsed, since he had no wallet or other ID, even though he was dressed pretty well. He's not a street person, that's for sure. No sign of a beating or any struggle. The cops took a few quick fingerprints and we might have some idea of who he is by tomorrow. He has a low white count, and some big cervical lymph nodes. A few in the axilla and groin as well. It's like mono, or cat scratch fever, maybe."

"Cat scratch fever? When does cat scratch fever make you comatose?"

"We don't have the toxicology back yet. His alcohol level is zero, but he may have barbiturates or heroin on board."

"Did you give him Narcan?" Narcan is the antidote for narcotic overdoses.

"Yeah, but that didn't do anything."

"Sort of rules out heroin . . . Here, here we go!" I pushed the needle forward and clear, watery fluid began to drip out. As I was switching collection tubes, the fluid splashed onto my face and eyes. I brushed it away with my coat sleeve. "This fluid looks pretty clear to me. No meningitis here."

"Thanks much, er"—she glanced quickly at my name tag—"Frank."

"No problem . . . (Try learning where the lumbar spine is next time) . . . Anytime at all. I'd get a stat gram stain on this stuff, anyway. He ain't like this for no reason. Maybe he has the Black Plague . . . maybe those groin nodes are really buboes." The intern blanched a bit. I was only half joking, since bubonic plague still exists in some parts of the country and, for the moment, we had no idea who Roger Doe was or where he called home.

I went back to my evening scut chores and forgot about the LP. Two hours later, the medical intern paged me with a curious bit of news.

"The Gram's stain," she said, referring to the microscopic examination of the fluid, "found many organisms resembling *Listeria monocytogenes.*"

"What the hell is that? I'm a surgeon, remember?"

"A gram-positive rod, a bacteria which causes meningitis, but only in alcoholics and in patients with cancer or leukemia."

"But he had clear fluid! And no pus!"

"I know. The official white count on the fluid was only three, normal. The glucose was a little low, but the fluid is teeming with bugs."

I thanked her and hung up. Why does someone have a rare meningitis, with no white cells in his spinal fluid? This was the healthiest sick guy I had ever seen.

Out of curiosity, I stopped into the medical ICU two days later to check on Roger Doe. He now had a name: William Bishop.

Forty-eight hours of intravenous antibiotics had done nothing to lighten his coma and he was now on a ventilator. The same intern who had botched his LP was standing by his bedside, along with a fellow from the infectious diseases department.

"Have you figured out what's wrong with Roger ... er, I mean, Mr. Bishop, yet? Oh, by the way"—I turned and addressed the infectious diseases fellow, a tall woman with horn-rimmed glasses—"I'm Frank, the neurosurgery resident who did his LP. The intern here told me he has *Listeria* meningitis."

The fellow nodded, her face dour.

"Well, we know several things. He does have *Listeria* meningitis; also has some form of pneumonia, we're not sure what type . . . he's getting an open lung biopsy this afternoon . . . and he has oral candidiasis." Candidiasis, called "thrush" in infants, is a yeast infection that almost never occurs in the mouths of adults unless they have had prolonged antibiotic therapy or have had their immune systems suppressed by disease or drug treatments.

"His family showed up from Ohio," the diminutive medical intern added, "but they haven't given us much useful information. It seems Mr. Bishop is a freelance artist and graphics designer who has been in town here for several weeks on a job. They haven't seen him in months, and he was the picture of health when he left Ohio. He doesn't do drugs, he doesn't smoke. In fact, he's a health nut. Whatever happened to him happened fairly quickly. He must have just passed out in the street one night, was robbed and left there to be picked up by police, who thought he was drunk. His tox screen was totally negative."

"I wouldn't say that they didn't provide us with any useful information," the fellow interjected. "I got two pieces of information that you didn't. He's a homosexual. And he's been to San Francisco."

The intern and I screwed up our faces in simultaneous puzzlement. I voiced what we were both thinking: "What difference does that make? I know—too much sourdough bread."

The fellow removed her glasses and spoke in low tones, as if she was about to convey top-secret information: "There are scattered reports coming out of cities with large populations of homosexual men, San Francisco in particular, concerning a new illness that afflicts only gay men. We've known for a while that this group is more prone to hepatitis B and a variety of other unusual things, such as gay bowel disease. Now, however, there seems to be a clustering of weird illnesses—Kaposi's sarcoma, pneumocystis pneumonia, candidiasis—occurring in homosexual men. Mr. Bishop fits that picture. He's homosexual, has been to San Francisco several times, has a low white count and several infections that occur only in people without competent immune systems. That seems to be the common denominator: immunodeficiency, or lack of normal immunity. There's no name for it yet."

"Is it contagious?" I asked with a shudder, thinking of the CSF I had cavalierly splashed about.

"No," replied the fellow. "At least we don't think so. Since only homosexual men are afflicted, it must be transmitted by something unique to their culture or their environments. One theory holds that it comes from the overuse of amyl nitrate, a drug used by homosexual men to heighten orgasm. Another hypothesis is that this is a virulent form of hepatitis B, but that seems far-fetched. Hepatitis B has been around a long time and has never been seen to cause anything like this. Some feel that geography matters, since the disease seems limited to the West Coast and to sections of Florida and the Caribbean—Haiti in particular."

I shrugged and left. Clearly not a neurosurgical problem. I found out later that Mr. Bishop had died of complications following his lung biopsy. The biopsy itself showed pneumocystis pneumonia. He became the first person reported to our local county health department with the strange new disease of gay men. Shortly thereafter, the illness got a name: AIDS.

* * *

Mr. Bishop's case faded from my memory, his name lost in the sea of names, faces, and diseases that a resident in a large medical center must deal with on a daily basis. Looking over my log book of operations and clinic visits, I once estimated that I took care of almost one thousand new patients each clinical year of my training. That number didn't include the William Bishops, those patients for whom we performed some bedside procedure or informal hallway consultation.

This is not to say that we forgot patients easily. While people in many occupations—bank tellers, food servers, mechanics, to name but a few—must deal with the public by the thousands annually, the interaction of physicians with the flux of humanity is unique. Bank tellers don't take personal histories. Food servers don't say you'll die within a year. For some reason, though, Mr. Bishop drifted out of my memory.

Years later, at the end of my chief residency year, I was speaking to one of the many insurance salespeople who dog us as we are about to finish our training. He was discussing disability policies and mentioned casually that I would have to be tested for cocaine and HIV before a policy could be issued. This was now standard for physicians. I shrugged it off: I don't use cocaine and I'm not gay . . . Then, suddenly, I remembered Mr. Bishop! The night of his LP came back to me in a rush, the few drops of spinal fluid that had splashed into my eyes were now oceans of contagion. In five years I hadn't developed AIDS, but the latency period between HIV infection and the full-blown clinical syndrome can be quite long.

How many other patients with HIV had I dipped my fingers into, whose bone dust had flown into my eyes and nostrils, whose spinal fluid had drenched my clothes? I had been up to my mask in bodily fluids during the blind era of the disease, when the virus was spreading but no test for it was available and few precautions were taken.

I took some comfort in the knowledge that our medical center was in an urban area with a very low prevalence of HIV. Nonetheless, I deferred getting tested for years, until I found it unavoidable. Mr. Bishop was never far from my mind during that long week which separated the drawing of the blood and the phone call informing me of the negative result.

But nothing would ever be the same again. The next person to roll into the ER could be the one who kills me.

6

Ailments Untreatable

At the university hospital, the days belonged to pain, the night to trauma. Our hospital was a "level I" trauma center, able to handle virtually any type of trauma except the most severe burn cases, which were diverted to the burn center across town.

There are two places where a body loses its human facade, where the trappings of personality, intelligence, and spirit fall away to reveal the Frankenstein mechanism of arteries, veins, and nerves beneath. One is the autopsy table. The other is the trauma room.

It was another night on call. I had retired to the spartan house-staff quarters on the hospital's uppermost floor to grab some sleep before facing the next day's overloaded operating schedule. The on-call room was little more than a hard bed and a loud phone. The doors didn't even lock—the legacy of a previous hospital administrator who feared that locked doors would mean too much sex among the house staff. The little that administrators do know about medicine must be garnered from daytime television. Soap opera M.D.'s may fornicate in the linen closets, but the average surgical house officer would more likely be caught sleeping there.

The emergency room awakened me at two in the

morning with word that an ambulance carrying an auto crash victim was pulling in. Before heading down to the ER, I stopped in the bathroom. Any patient too ill to wait for me to pee was likely to die with or without my help.

I entered the trauma room just as a pale and bloodied young woman was being lifted from the ambulance stretcher onto the trauma room gurney. She was strapped to a "backboard," a wooden platform used to immobilize the entire spine. A paramedic in a blue jumpsuit droned her report to all within earshot: "Caucasian female, age twenty-two . . . unrestrained passenger in a car traveling at high rate of speed down Bigelow Boulevard. The car crossed the center line and collided with another vehicle. Victim was found awake but incoherent outside of the vehicle. Blood pressure 100 over 60, pulse 125. An open laceration in the right frontal parietal area was packed to stop bleeding. Large blood loss was apparent at the scene. No obvious limb fractures or deformities were noted. The patient moves all four extremities spontaneously, but follows no commands. . . ."

Fearing that more trouble was on the way, I asked the paramedic what had happened to the other victims of the crash.

"Two people in the other car were taken to Mercy Hospital," she replied, adding under her breath, "and the driver of her vehicle was dead at the scene. We pronounced him and called a coroner's ambulance."

"You pronounced him?" I asked with mock indignation. Officially, only a licensed physician can make the pronouncement of death.

"It doesn't take an M.D. to know when a headless guy is dead," she answered with a slight smile. I still had a lot to learn about street trauma. The paramedic crew retired to the front desk to complete their reports and await the return of their backboard.

Nurses quickly cut the clothes from the injured woman's arms and torso. Until the extent of spinal injury is known, excessive movement of the patient is unwise and the more civil methods of removing clothing are too dangerous. For those with minor injuries, watching a beloved sweater being shorn from their bodies like fleece from a sheep can be more traumatizing than their accidents. The victim's lower body was encased in a blue MAST suit, a comical set of inflatable pantaloons used to force blood from the expendable legs into the not-so-expendable head.

I donned a pair of latex gloves and removed the gauze pads the paramedics had stuffed into the head wound. Pulling away blood-caked hair, I separated the edges of the lacerated scalp. The wound was eight or ten inches in length and filled with road dirt and fragments of windshield glass. The glistening ivory surface of the skull showed; a jagged fracture ran parallel to the laceration. Pink, macerated brain tissue the consistency of toothpaste leaked from the fracture line.

The Edwin Smith papyrus, an ancient Egyptian medical text dating back to 1700 B.C., declared that any patient with brain tissue oozing from a skull fracture had "an ailment untreatable." Nearly four thousand years of medical progress had not disproved this grim prognosis.

I ruffled through the papers stuffed under the backboard, searching for her first name . . . Shirley. Under normal circumstances I would never address a new patient by her first name. Such uninvited familiarity is the province of car salesmen, not physicians, but a severely head injured patient requires a less polite approach.

A first name is the most durable lifeline to the outside world, the first word recognized and the last word forgotten. When a dementing illness erases our awareness of home, spouse, and children, we will still answer to our first name. A first name can pierce the delirious fog of head trauma faster than any other word. Leaning close to her face, I smelled her alcohol-laden blood—a nauseating aroma unique to emergency rooms.

"Shirley," I spoke directly into her ear. She slowly opened her eyes.

"Yes?" she answered, her voice muffled by the green plastic oxygen mask draped over her mouth.

"Shirley, my name is Frank. You've been in a car accident and you're in the hospital. I don't think you have been badly hurt, but we have to do a bunch of things here. It's going to be a long night. Can you wiggle your toes and fingers for me?"

After a brief delay she obeyed, feebly, and then closed her eyes again. Although I was encouraged that she was not unconscious, I remained skeptical about her chances for survival. I had seen "talk and die" patients before, those who have a short period of wakefulness followed by a slow descent into coma and brain death. Just as a sprained ankle may not bruise and swell until hours after being twisted, the injured brain may not succumb to edema until several hours after a lethal impact.

The skull is a best friend and worst enemy to the gelatinous organ within. During normal daily activities, the brain sways to and fro in a watery sea of spinal fluid, tethered to the bone by small veins. During rapid acceleration and deceleration, such as during a car crash or during the vigorous "shaking" of a crying infant (one of the leading causes of infant murders), the brain slams into the skull and rips loose from its venous moorings. Blood oozes from the torn veins, forming compressive clots known as subdural hematomas, while edema fluid collects in the bruised areas of the brain. Trapped within the skull's bony confines, the swelling brain chokes off its own blood supply and strangulates. In a trauma, the skull turns from a brain's protector to its murderer, and, finally, to its coffin.

The surgeon can intervene by removing blood clots and giving drugs to reduce brain swelling, but the damage is often irreversible. Surgeons in Japan tried removing the top of the skull in these patients, allowing injured brains unlimited space in which to swell. The skull's "lid" was stored temporarily in a refrigerator, to be replaced when the swelling subsided. In some cases, unfortunately, the brain swelled to monstrous proportions, making the patient's head look like something from a bad science-fiction movie. The patients died anyway and the practice has been abandoned.

In desperate cases, large sections of the brain can be hacked away to make room for more swelling—a kamikaze strategy. In a macabre sense, Shirley was performing this type of surgery upon herself by squeezing her swollen brain tissue through the open skull fracture. The continuous decompression of dead, liquefied brain matter from her wound may have been the only thing keeping her alive at the moment.

"Shirley, you have a cut on your head from the windshield and this young doctor is going to put some stitches in your head." I instructed the general surgery intern to suture the laceration using a quick layer of running nylon. Since I was likely to reopen the wound in the operating room in a few hours, a cosmetic closure was unnecessary. "It doesn't have to be a Rembrandt; just stop the bleeding. And try to keep her hair out of the wound." He grimaced at the sight of a growing mound of brain exuding from the wound. I wiped it away with a gauze sponge. "Memories of third grade," I whispered, "but don't let it bother you; she won't miss it."

Bill, the senior surgical resident, examined the woman's chest and abdomen while his junior residents performed other standard chores: drawing blood samples for the lab, inserting large intravenous lines, feeling along her arms and legs for any palpable fractures or lacerations, debriding the skin of dirt and glass.

"Type and cross her for six units of blood," Bill instructed a trauma nurse, "and see if they can send down some type O in case she crashes. What's her pressure now?"

"Ninety over sixty."

"Force in another liter of lactated Ringer's as fast as you can and get the X-ray people in here."

I called the CT technician to let him know that we needed an urgent brain scan. A physician must wake up a lot of people in the middle of the night and attempt to engage them in meaningful conversation.

"Hello," a dreamy voice answered.

"Are you the CT technician on call?"

"Hello?"

"IS THIS THE CT TECH ON CALL?"

There was a pause and the rustling of bedsheets. *Christ, I thought, he's falling asleep.* The previous month, a tech had dropped the phone on the floor while I was talking to her and gone back to sleep. I had to send the police to get her.

". . . Uh, is this the hospital?" The tech was barely conscious.

"No," I replied, "it's Ed McMahon calling you from Publisher's Clearinghouse. You have just won one million dollars. And, by the way, I've got a trauma here in the ER and I need a scan now."

"OK."

It wasn't a convincing okay, more like the okay of someone who was slipping back into slumberland, to awake in four hours wondering if the hospital had really called or if he'd just had a nightmare. I called again ten minutes later and was informed by his irate wife that he indeed was on his way.

Perhaps I was a little rude, but I didn't care. I now knew how James Bond must feel when he thinks he's saving the world from certain destruction. Politeness and civility are sacrificed without a trace of guilt. As the earth teeters on the brink of nuclear holocaust, Bond runs through a crowded airport knocking people flat, kicking over their luggage and spilling their drinks—all without so much as an "Excuse me." He's not rude; he's a hero on a mission. He can grab people by the throat, hold a gun to their heads—anything to get the job done. I can say: "Get your ass out of bed and scan this lady BEFORE SHE DIES." In the end, all is allowed, all is forgiven. We do what we have to do. Results, not effort.

Shirley's blood pressure began to rise and stabilize. The intern had finished closing her scalp and the X-ray technicians were setting up to take chest, neck, and abdominal films.

"Shirley, are you still there?" I asked.

"Yes, but my head hurts. Am I going to die?"

"No. Too much paperwork if you die. We're going to take some X-rays films."

"How's Jack? I want to see him."

"Uhmmm . . . he's not here right now. They took him someplace else." A diplomatic response. She was in no condition to learn that her friend had been guillotined. Bill and I retreated to the small coffee lounge, where we feasted on a box of vanilla wafers stamped "For Institutional Use Only." I had gained twenty pounds in three months on the boss's service from eating vanilla wafers washed down with chocolate milk and was becoming an "institution" myself, at least in terms of body habitus. The coffee was a day old, but we drank it anyway for its medicinal properties.

"This is just fucking great," Bill complained. "I have a Whipple to do tomorrow and I'm going to be totally fried. We get a Whipple about twice a year." An operation for pancreatic cancer, the complicated Whipple procedure was something that the general surgery residents slather over.

"At least you may be able to go back to bed soon," I countered, "but she's got the gray matter coming out of her head. She's going to need a craniotomy if she doesn't croak first. And the boss has all four of our OR's booked at seven-thirty. If he gets bumped by this case he'll blow a fuse."

I glanced at my watch. It was now three-thirty. My mind turned to those bureaucratic dilemmas which consume so much of a resident's time and energy. There was no way I was going to get Shirley scanned and complete a craniotomy fast enough to avoid delaying the boss in one of his rooms. Tomorrow was his squash day, too. If he wasn't done by noon it would be me who'd need a craniotomy. And who was going to cover my room if I was in the OR with this case? I could put the intern in my room, but that would piss off the boss. He'd go bananas on the intern, and then the intern would hate me for the rest of his neurosurgery rotation. Tuesday was always our biggest day. Why did these cases always roll in on Monday night? Who went out drinking and driving on a Monday night?

I could ask anesthesia for a fifth neurosurgery room. I could ask Mother Teresa for a date, too; the answer would be the same. I glanced over the OR schedule tacked to the bulletin board. Four heart rooms, four ortho rooms, four neuro rooms ... it was hopeless. They'd never give us five rooms. I had to either bump one of the boss's cases to a later time or cancel one altogether. I pulled out my patient list, called the neuro nursing station, and spoke to Karen, the night charge nurse.

"Karen, this is Frank. Is there any excuse for canceling one of the seven-thirty cases tomorrow, like a fever, a low potassium—anything?"

"Let me look." There was a pause as she went off to review the charts. "Well," Karen returned, flipping pages, "Mr. Jamieson's potassium is 3.5."

"Not low enough."

"How about Mrs. Bates, the hemifacial spasm," Karen continued, "her temp at midnight was 99.7."

"Not high enough. Has everyone signed consents? Doesn't anyone have any doubts? Maybe someone needs an extra day to think about their surgery? It is brain surgery, after all."

"No chance. These are the boss's patients, remember?"

"Yeah, right. If you think of anything let me know. I have a trauma down here who is about to fuck with our elective schedule."

I crammed my patient sheets back into my coat pocket, finished my coffee, and returned to the trauma room, where Bill was already reviewing the chest film.

"Her mediastinum is a tad wide," he murmured to me. "She'll need an aortogram."

The aorta, a gargantuan artery which carries blood from the heart, descends between the two lungs on its way to the abdomen in a chest space called the mediastinum. In the mediastinum, the aorta is tethered by a short ligament called the ductus, the remnant of the embryonic artery which shunts blood away from our fluid-filled fetal lungs. In the rapid deceleration of a car crash, the ductus acts as the aorta's seat belt, restraining the jumbo artery's midsection while the rest of it continues to move forward at great speed. In a violent crash, even a young and resilient aorta can tear and leak blood into the mediastinum, widening the space around the heart as seen on chest X rays. A leaking aorta, like a leaking dam, can burst at any time. For Shirley, an aortic tear meant that her great blood vessel would have to be replaced with a Teflon tube before a terminal hemorrhage occurred.

Shirley was now the typical "multiple" trauma. With at least two of her vital organs in need of surgical repair, we had to decide which organ took priority. Was it better to have a new Teflon aorta transmitting blood to a worthless brain, or a good brain in a body dead from aortic rupture? We hadn't even tapped her belly—what surprises lurked there?

Although it was possible to operate on the brain and

chest simultaneously, the thoracic surgeons would have to "thin" Shirley's blood with the anticoagulant drug heparin during the time her damaged aorta was clamped. Otherwise, the stagnant, nonflowing blood would clot off in her aorta. Anticoagulation made brain surgery out of the question. The brain is the bloodiest organ in the body, and any attempt to manipulate it without the body's clotting mechanisms in full working order would be a lethal exercise. I decided that if she needed both brain and chest operations, they would have to be done separately. I just hoped her belly tap was clean.

A belly tap is made just below the navel: a thin tube is inserted into the abdominal cavity through a tiny incision. Sterile saline is injected, swished around, and aspirated. If the fluid returns tinged with blood, then a spleen rupture or liver laceration is likely. Yellow, turbid fluid indicates a bowel injury. A junior surgical resident began painting Shirley's abdomen with orange Betadine solution, while a nurse unwrapped a belly tap kit and placed it on the Mayo stand beside him.

"Shirley, are you still there?" I asked.

"Yes."

She was sleepier, more distant. Her left hand grasp was weaker. Worrisome. Her head was going bad faster than I had planned. The scanner people would be here soon. Bill was on the phone to the angio people, arranging a dye test to look for the suspected leak in Shirley's aorta. With the possibility of a growing intracranial clot, however, she might not last the one or two hours necessary for an aortic angiogram. I would be forced to take her to the OR without it. Of course, Bill would object and we would have one of our frequent fights over which organ system needed attention first.

I reached Dr. Sakren, the attending neurosurgeon on call, and notified him of the situation. His political weight might bully the thoracic surgeons into letting us work first. Sakren was less than enthusiastic—"Call me back if you really need me": code language for "Deal with it yourself, I'm sleeping." Thanks a bunch.

That's why people go to university centers: in search of first-year neurosurgical residents to make their life-and-death decisions for them. I was hoping for more moral support from the attending, but calling him again could be construed as unmanly. In a neurosurgical residency, one of the last male-dominated bastions of medicine, looking unmanly is almost as bad as looking lazy. I let him sleep.

Shirley's belly-tap fluid came back crystal clear—the abdominal organs had escaped major damage. Had Shirley been wearing her seat belt, her injuries would have been reversed. Instead of shattering the windshield with her head when ejecting from the car, she would have crushed her lower abdomen against the belt, perhaps lacerating her small intestine. In any violent collision, something in the body must take the impact force, something must give. Intestines can be repaired. Fixing the brain is much harder.

The rest of Shirley's X rays had been developed and delivered to the trauma room. The neck and lower-back films disclosed no fractures or dislocations. I released the straps on her bulky vinyl cervical collar and allowed her to be moved from the backboard. The board was quickly wiped clean and returned to the paramedic crew, who had finished their paperwork and were anxious to get back on the road.

I told the operating room that an emergency craniotomy was brewing, they should set up a brain instrument tray. The night charge nurse gave me the usual grief about the liver transplant that was still going on, the heart patient who was oozing from his chest tubes and might have to "come back," the open fracture from three hours ago that ortho was still trying to get on the schedule. It was the same story every night I tried to do a case.

"Don't the transplant people ever work during the day? What are they, vampires? Look, I don't really care what's happening up there; just set up a room now." That James Bond feeling again.

"All right, we'll set up in one of your morning rooms. You'll have to bump one of Abramowitz's seven-thirty retromastoids." There was a "nyah-nyah" tone in her voice. She knew that bumping his cases carried a risk of castration.

"Can't you put me in one of the general surgery rooms? We'll be out by nine or nine-thirty, I promise." Really, Mother Teresa, you'll have a wonderful time ... I know a place, great Indian food. . . .

"No way. Don't get greedy. With the backup of cases from last night, you're lucky we don't take away another one of your rooms, too, so be thankful you still have four start times. What time will you be up?"

"The scanner people should be here soon. I guess thirty minutes." It was actually going to take an hour or more to get to the OR, but they didn't need to know that.

Bill had overheard my conversation. "What about my aortogram?"

"Sure, Bill, if there's time." (No way, my friend. Brains first, big bloody hoses second.)

"We have to make time."

"If the angio people are here, we'll take her right from CT to the angio suite, and then to the OR. But she needs a craniotomy before she gets her chest cracked." No matter what the scan showed, the skull fracture would have to be cleaned out and any bone fragments or hair driven into the brain removed.

"Fine." Bill seemed satisfied with the compromise. "But I want to see that aortogram. If she's dissecting we have to do that as soon as you're through."

True enough, but an aortic dissection would really blow my OR schedule to hell. To get a new aorta, Shirley would be in the neuro room until two or three in the afternoon, meaning that two or more of our elective patients would have to be canceled outright, not just delayed. Holy shit! I didn't even want to think about that. I pulled out my patient sheet again. Who would it be? The Italian businessman who'd flown halfway around the world for his operation? Nope, he stays on the schedule. The wife of the director of a major metropolitan opera company? Abramowitz had some big hitters in the day's lineup. No one would go quietly. Please, Shirley, have a good aorta.

I suddenly felt very tired. The next day's work loomed ahead. I could envision each burr hole I would have to drill, each scalp stitch I would have to place, each small brain bleeder I would have to coagulate. Hundreds of tiny motions and I didn't feel like doing any goddamned one of them.

The trauma room's intercom buzzed. "The patient's parents are in the waiting room," the desk clerk informed us. As bad as I thought my night was, this family's night was going to be worse. To me, she was as much a bureaucratic nuisance as she was a patient. To them, she was a first step, a first word, a first bicycle, a first date. Decades of their lives, a fond tapestry woven of birthday parties, summer vacations, proms, and graduations, was shredding apart in our ER. The baby they'd tossed into the air now dripped her brains into four-by-four gauze sponges. Bill and I went out to talk with them. Medicine at its ugliest.

The middle-aged couple remained sniffly but stalwart throughout our presentation. Bill discussed the need for a dye test to check the main artery in her body and the possibility that the artery might have to be repaired surgically. I discussed the nature of her head injury and obtained their consent for the brain surgery. They asked the usual questions about her chances for meaningful survival, what she would be like, had her face been badly damaged, and could they see her before she went to surgery. I dodged the recovery issue, stressing that she had suffered no obvious cosmetic damage and was not in severe pain. Doctors are like politicians: we stress the good things. Since we were doing all we could as rapidly as we could, I doubted that there would be time for her parents to talk with Shirley before she went to the scanner.

For her family, this was a nightmare of biblical proportions. Pulled from a sound sleep into a dim ER waiting room and forced to listen to the planned dissection of their daughter, these poor people could not have been encouraged by our appearance. With our five o'clock shadows, uncombed hair, and iodine-stained lab jackets, we must have looked like high school students to them, right down to our soiled tennis shoes.

I put my hand on the mother's shoulder, saying that I would be back when I knew more. We returned to the trauma room. The heavy metal door clanked shut, sealing off the waiting room from our brightly lit inner sanctum. A nurse was disconnecting Shirley's heart electrodes from the wall monitor and hooking them to a portable monitor/defibrillator perched on the end of her bed. A respiratory technician attached Shirley's oxygen mask to a small green tank. The scanner was ready and they were preparing her to be transported from the ER.

The scanners were in the adjoining children's hospital, one flight up and about two hundred yards away from the trauma room. The operating rooms were yet another flight up, and another two hundred yards away from the scanners. When transporting an unstable patient, even a brief elevator ride and short roll down a hallway can be an unsettling experience. Surgeons feel comfortable only in the operating room. The operating room sits in a virtual sea of specialized instruments, resuscitation equipment, and anesthesia expertise. Field trips to radiology were like moon walks, the patient tethered to a precarious lifeline of battery-powered monitors and small scuba tanks of oxygen, far from an anesthesiologist and a good instrument set.

"What's her pressure doing?" Bill asked.

"Ninety over fifty," replied a nurse.

"I'm not happy about transporting her until we hang some blood. Is there blood in the room?"

I examined Shirley again. Brain matter still oozed from the sutured scalp laceration. "Wiggle your toes." This time she wiggled only the toes of her right foot. "Wiggle the toes of your left foot." Again the right foot. She was developing some paralysis on her left side. At this rate, it was only a matter of time before she started talking about bright lights beckoning her to "cross over to the other side," or some other hallucination common to dying brains.

"We need to scan her," I told Bill.

"The blood's here," he argued back. "It'll take just five minutes to hang a unit on a pump bag. Her hematocrit's only twenty-eight, she's had seven liters of fluid, and her pressure's falling again."

"What's happening to me?" Shirley cried suddenly as she reached up to pull the oxygen mask away with her remaining good arm. Jan, one of the night nurses, grabbed her arm and told her to relax.

"But I can't breathe!" she cried hoarsely as she began to struggle with the nurse, jerking with her right arm and twisting her head grotesquely from side to side. I looked at the portable heart monitor. Her heart rate, which had been about 120 for the last hour, had jumped to 190.

"Pressure," Bill ordered.

"Seventy over palp."

"Get anesthesia, stat. She's going to need a tube. And get me a chest tray and call the cardiothoracic fellow down here."

I knew what Bill was thinking. Shirley was no longer losing blood from her scalp and her belly tap showed no evidence of abdominal bleeding. The falling pressure must be due to blood escaping from the rending aorta in her chest. Her inability to breathe was a sign that her chest was filling with blood, crowding her lungs. Her heart was pumping furiously to make up for the decreased blood volume. She was "shocking out." Opening her chest and clamping her aorta right there might be her only chance of survival. Anesthesia would have to insert an endotracheal tube and put her to sleep. If they didn't arrive in time, Bill would do it with her awake.

Nurses and aides darted from other ER rooms, helping to ferry messages to the front desk. In addition to the anesthesiologist and cardiothoracic fellow, the attending trauma surgeon was notified, and the operating room. Two floors up, the OR technicians began putting away the cranial drills and brain retractors and began setting up the heart-lung machine and chest instruments. An ER medical resident came in and helped Bill insert another IV line. One of the other senior surgical residents on call had arrived and was unwrapping the ER chest tray and preparing some chest tubes, long plastic hoses that are inserted into the chest to drain blood and air. The doors to the other ER rooms were closed to shield the few other patients from the unfolding spectacle.

I remained at the head of her bed. Shirley's eyes were wide open, her pupils unequal. She was panting in brief, labored breaths; her color had turned ashen. Jan handed me an Ambu bag, a device used to assist the patient's breathing. I removed the oxygen mask and firmly pressed the Ambu over her mouth, squeezing the bag hard to drive in air. "I'm dying, I'm dying," she gasped between squeezes.

She was right, she most certainly was dying. We have an innate ability to tell when something is lethally awry in our bodies. My father had chest pains for years before his first heart attack, but we could tell from his face on the morning of that first attack that this pain was different. There was panic in his eyes. Physicians don't get concerned about patients' asking if they are going to die, but when a patient blurts out "I'm dying!" we know that this is often an accurate prediction.

The nurse-anesthetist and anesthesiologist came bustling into the room carrying a large tackle box full of laryngoscopes, endotracheal tubes, and anesthetic drugs. The nurse-anesthetist displaced me at the head of the bed and began squeezing the Ambu bag. "I can't ventilate her," she said to the anesthesiologist. He quickly handed her a laryngoscope, which she snapped open like a switch blade. It had a long silver spatula with a light at the tip, which she inserted into Shirley's mouth. At the same time, the anesthesiologist injected a combination of curare-like drugs and narcotics into one of Shirley's many intravenous lines. These drugs would paralyze and sedate her so that she would not fight the efforts to breathe for her.

The nurse-anesthetist cocked Shirley's head back and pushed the steel blade deep into her throat, lifting her tongue away so that the entrance to her windpipe could be seen. Shirley coughed and retched violently on the scope's blade, straining against the cloth restraints that tied her right arm and leg to the stretcher. The curare finally took effect and Shirley's struggling ceased. "I see the cords. Give me a tube." The anesthetist was staring at Shirley's vocal cords. She was handed a clear plastic tube coated with petroleum jelly, which she slipped between the vocal cords into Shirley's windpipe.

I stepped out of the room and watched from the hallway. Over a dozen people filled the small room now, and I was the most dispensable of the lot. Since Shirley was under general anesthesia, I could no longer follow her brain function. Her skin color deteriorated further, to the pasty yellow-blue hue of a cadaver. "Pressure fifty over palp." The EKG monitor showed runs of ventricular tachycardia, the heart's equivalent of "throwing a rod" from being pushed too hard. Her tank was running dry.

Bill and the cardiothoracic fellow, who had just darted in, took off their lab coats and put on sterile gloves as the intern poured a bottle of Betadine onto Shirley's exposed chest. The respiratory therapist, a large man with muscular forearms, attached the Ambu bag to the endotracheal tube and squeezed hard. Even with the tube in place, his strong hands could barely force air into Shirley's collapsing lungs.

I knew this flurry of activity was nothing but a dance of death for poor Shirley. Her aorta had burst, spilling blood into her chest. Like a jetliner with its hydraulics destroyed, her body was still flying but had no hope of landing safely. In a few minutes her life was going to come thundering to the ground in ER room eight.

Bill plunged a number 10 scalpel blade to the hilt in her chest wall and cleaved a twelve-inch window under the left breast. As he entered the pleura, the thick leathery covering of the lung, a huge glob of clotted blood slithered out and splattered to the floor. The cardiothoracic fellow jammed a rib spreader into the wound and cranked it open, splaying open the chest cavity as rib bones cracked and popped. I continued to observe for a while as the two men muttered to each other, passing their arms, bloodstained to the elbow, in and out of the chest wound. They held back the foamy pink lung as they probed with long metal clamps and needle holders. The thin, purple blood continued to flow unchecked out of the wound and onto their clothes and shoes.

Shirley's blood pressure collapsed. Her tracing on the monitor writhed chaotically as the heart's rhythm degenerated into fruitless quivering and fibrillations. An alarm sounded from the monitor—it was the sound of my OR schedule becoming whole again. The cardiothoracic fellow reached deep into the chest and grabbed the heart, manually massaging the flaccid ventricles. "Empty," was his simple pronouncement. She was gone. He withdrew his arm, removed his gloves, and went to the sink to wash.

"Will you talk with the family?" I called in to Bill, who nodded grimly as he continued to stare into Shirley's chest. Thank God. I could just imagine those poor people sitting out there watching the parade of people rushing into the ER. I'd told her mother I would be back. I'd lied. This was a trauma surgery death, not mine. The general surgeons could play the grim reaper on this one.

In the OR, the chest instruments were being repacked and the room readied once more for Dr. Abramowitz's first patient. An irate CT technician, his night disturbed for no good purpose, was shutting down his computer. Unused blood was packed up and trundled back to the central blood bank to await the next disaster. The angio people were going home. The small medical army drafted for this war was quickly demobilized. The cleanup people were summoned. Bill assigned the hapless intern the task of closing the dead woman's chest. "It doesn't have to be a Rembrandt."

On this night I had the singular honors of hearing a woman's last words, of denying her parents the right to see her alive one last time, and of permitting her to die believing that her boyfriend was still alive. Eight floors up, seven people on the neurosurgical OR schedule were sleeping, unaware that, for a few hours, I had been rearranging their futures in my head. As it turned out, their surgeries would go on as planned and the boss would play his squash.

7

Surgical Psychopaths

The trauma experiences hardened me to death and the pain patients made me cynical about suffering. I felt my personality slipping away during this arduous process of becoming "one of them." Clinical cases no longer evoked the strong emotions they once had. The humiliation of that first unsuccessful nasogastric tube, the panic as B.G.'s fingers died at my command—I looked back upon such mushy feelings with a bemused nostalgia, like a worldly playboy reminiscing about the naive crush on his sixth-grade teacher.

Yet, my emotional numbness was still only partial. I hadn't progressed to the status of a true surgical psychopath, wherein one's humanity is placed under general anesthesia. I first learned about surgical psychopathy from the sad case of a man named Andy.

Life had been unkind to Andy from the very beginning. His troubles started before his conception, with a chromosome blunder within the developing eggs of his mother's ovaries. The blueprint for a human body resides in its chromosomes, our molecular heirlooms, which consist of tightly coiled bundles of DNA passed from generation to generation. As the human egg and sperm are formed, chromosomes are shuffled like poker cards as nature tries to deal the best hand to our offspring. In Andy's case, the shuffled DNA deck dealt him a loser.

We're supposed to possess forty-six chromosomes: twenty-two pairs of non-sex chromosomes, and two sex chromosomes consisting of either two X's (in women) or an X and a Y (in men). Each parent donates half of the total pool of a child's genetic material: one sex chromosome and one each of the twenty-two different non-sex chromosomes.

Because of a foul-up in making the egg that would become Andy, his mother gave him not one but two copies of chromosome 21. Since one chromosome 21 was also contributed by his father, Andy thus inherited three, not the normal two, copies of chromosome 21's DNA blueprints, a condition called trisomy 21.

This mistake most commonly occurs during the process of meiosis, when the mother's chromosomes are packaged into eggs for dispersion to her children, although the error can occur in other ways as well. The likelihood of producing a trisomy egg increases as the ovaries age and the egg-making machinery becomes senile, misplacing chromosomes as an octogenarian might misplace eyeglasses.

DNA has been called the currency of life. Unlike money, however, it *is* possible to have too much DNA. Trisomy 21 is associated with varying degrees of mental retardation, a high incidence of congenital heart defects, and an increased chance of childhood leukemia. Decades ago, those afflicted with trisomy 21 were called "mongoloids" because of the thick eyelid folds which give trisomies a vaguely Oriental appearance. This offensive label was replaced with the more medical-sounding "Down syndrome." Some argued that the late Dr. Down should not be so eponymously rewarded. Down's critics charge that he was a racist who believed that trisomy 21 victims actually were "inferior" Mongolians who appeared sporadically in the Western population. The technical term "trisomy 21" is now most commonly used.

In addition to trisomy 21, Andy was also afflicted with multiple head and neck abnormalities. His ear canals were small and misshapen, making him deaf from birth. A low hairline sat barely an inch above his wide-set eyes. Malformed vocal cords rendered him mute. Unfortunately, this simultaneous clustering of genetic defects is not rare. The opposite situation, people with nothing but stellar genes, also occurs. Who hasn't known someone born with a royal flush of genes, the high school beauty queen who is class valedictorian and captain of the swim team as well? But alas, for each genetic success story, there is an Andy.

Andy had a social disadvantage as well: he was born in the 1930s, when special education for disabled children was not widely available. Andy *did* have several things going for him. He was born to loving parents who reared him at home when institutionalizing trisomy victims was the norm. Moreover, he had been spared the ravages of trisomy-related heart defects, and he even had a respectable IQ of 80.

Though he never went to mainstream schools, he still managed to learn sign language, as well as how to read a little. He was emotionally untroubled, passing his time doing odd jobs as they became available.

Andy eventually settled into a job as the janitor of his local Catholic church, where he would spend hours polishing the hardwood pews. He particularly enjoyed preparing the church for holidays. As the decades passed, the task of putting up the decorations for Easter and Christmas became entirely his own, a responsibility he cherished. Andy became the bedrock of St. Mary's, a fixture at Mass, a benevolent Buddha at summer bazaars and spaghetti dinners. Pastors came and went, but Andy stayed.

As years passed, he became increasingly obese, smoked heavily, and developed diabetes and high blood pressure. One day shortly after his forty-fifth birthday, he went suddenly blind in his right eye from a diabetic retinal hemorrhage, making his left eye his sole link to the world. Timely laser surgery forestalled blindness in that good eye, but Andy knew his vision was failing and he subsequently battled bouts of depression. Despite his health problems, he was at the church shortly after dawn seven days a week.

One humid morning in the summer of Andy's forty-seventh year, his mother was awakened by the sound of retching in the downstairs bathroom. She found her only child seated by the toilet holding his large head in his hands and rocking slowly back and forth. His broad face was chalklike and glistening with cold sweat. He signed, "I'm sick," and "Help me, Mom" repeatedly before slumping onto his side, unconscious.

I was shooting pool in the residents' recreational area on the hospital's tenth floor when my pager went off, disturbing a surprisingly quiet Saturday afternoon. The beeper display read "1667." A call from the outside. Bad news.

I dialed the extension and was connected to an ER nurse at Suburban Hospital.

"Please hold for Dr. Najarian."

During the long wait my mind conjured up all sorts of grim possibilities lurking for me in the Suburban ER. Was it one of the pain patients? A head trauma? A bleed?

"Hello, who am I speaking to?" the voice finally came.

"Vertosick," I replied dryly, "neurosurgery resident."

"I have a mongoloid in his late forties, history of hypertension, comes in this morning lethargic, found down in his bathroom by his mother after vomiting times one. BP is 230 over 120, pulse fifty-five. He's deaf and mute, but can communicate with sign language with his mother as interpreter. He's complaining of a headache, has no focal deficits. Our CT scanner is down and we'd like to transport him. I think he has a hypertensive bleed."

"Is he on any meds?" I pulled out a crumpled note card and began jotting down information.

"Inderal, Dyazide. He's allergic to penicillin. He's also diabetic, but not being treated as far as I can tell. He's got partial blindness, I don't know what from—perhaps from retinopathy."

"Do I have this right—he has Down syndrome, he's deaf, he's partially blind, he can't speak, and he has a bleed?" Wow. This was going to be a long weekend.

"Yeah, and he lives at home with his parents, who look about a thousand years old. Still, they seem in better shape than he is."

"What's his name?"

There was a pause as Dr. Najarian searched his

notes. It's amazing how physicians can remember blood pressures, medications, and allergies, but never something as trivial as a name.

"Andy . . . Andy Wood."

"Go ahead and send him now. By helicopter." End of conversation.

I racked up the balls again. It would take several hours for the helicopter to arrive.

At 5 P.M. the med flight crew rolled into the emergency room with Andy. Forewarned, I was in the ER when the helicopter team wheeled him into the exam room. Even though he was wrapped in a scarlet blanket, Andy's obesity was obvious. His eyes were covered with a white washcloth, and an oxygen mask clung loosely to his lower face. His mouth was hanging open, his oversized tongue protruding in typical trisomy fashion.

"Is he awake?" I asked one of the flight nurses.

"Yeah," he replied, "but I guess you know he's deaf and mute. His mother says that you can write him notes and he'll write back, but he won't keep his eyes open long enough to read anything."

"How's his pressure?"

"Still high, about 160 or 190. He got some Aldomet prior to leaving, and some Lasix and Decadron."

He would need an arterial line and a nitroprusside drip to keep his blood pressure from blowing his brain into the next room.

"Anybody know where his parents are?" I yelled into the room.

"They're driving down, I think," another one of the flight nurses volunteered, "but I don't know when they'll get here."

I removed the washcloth from Andy's face. He winced at the glaring ER light and promptly snatched the cloth from my hand and returned it to his face. Photophobia; the light bothered him. I reached behind his clammy neck and began flexing his head up and down. His arm shot out rapidly to stop me and he made a guttural, almost inhuman, noise. His neck was stiff and sore. Maybe this wasn't a simple hypertensive bleed. I began to think Andy had suffered a subarachnoid hemorrhage, or SAH.

SAH results from the rupturing of cerebral aneurysms, saccular outpouchings that can occur on the large arteries at the base of the brain. After decades of weathering the incessant pounding of blood, arteries can develop small weaknesses. The weaknesses slowly sprout into thin-walled blebs, similar to the balloonlike outgrowths that form on old inner tubes.

Like the ER doctor, I initially believed that Andy had suffered a hypertensive bleed, an event quite different from SAH. Hypertensive bleeds are not caused by aneurysms on large arteries. They arise instead from tiny arteries that simply "pop" when the blood pressure becomes too great. Hypertensive bleeds occur deep within the brain and, although they can render a patient paralyzed, are rarely fatal. SAH, on the other hand, is quite frequently lethal.

Even though the bleeding during an SAH can be slight and doesn't damage the brain substance directly, it is a devastating event. A person may silently harbor an aneurysm for years until some stress, such as sexual intercourse, lifting a heavy box, or simply having a violent sneeze, sends a pulse wave of blood pressure that splits the fragile aneurysm sac, spilling a torrent of arterial blood into the space between the brain and the skull. This region is called the "subarachnoid space" because it is below the arachnoid, a cottony substance which covers the brain and which derives its name from its close resemblance to a spider's web.

The victim of an SAH is felled immediately by a "thunderclap" headache, as if shot by a gun. Vomiting may occur. The body reacts quickly to stem the hemorrhage by sending the blood vessels feeding the aneurysm into spasm, temporarily closing them off. Arterial spasm is the body's natural defense against hemorrhage—it's what allows a Kansas farmboy the time to pick up his arm after it has been amputated by a threshing machine and run for help without bleeding to death.

An arm can go hours without blood and survive. The brain's survival time without oxygen is three minutes. Several minutes after a brain aneurysm ruptures, the feeding arteries are compelled to reopen by chemical signals from the starving brain tissue. If a sufficient protective clot has not formed over the rent in the aneurysm's wall, the bleeding will resume, with lethal results. If the arteries don't reopen at all, bleeding will cease but large areas of the brain will die, or "stroke," with resulting paralysis or coma.

During the first minutes after SAH, the patient's life teeters on a precipice. The brain's life-sustaining arteries seek to maintain a level of blood flow which prevents stroke but which will not blow open the aneurysmal tear. Within a two- or three-cubic-centimeter area beneath the ailing brain, biochemical processes a billion years in the making converge in a matter of milliseconds—processes such as blood coagulation, already ancient when the dinosaurs roamed. For almost half the victims of SAH, the body's efforts to save itself are in vain—death follows in days, even hours.

I notified the surgical intensive-care unit that Andy had arrived. We then transferred him quickly to a transport cart. There was little we could do for him in the emergency room, and the faster we got him into the more relaxed environment of a hospital bed, the better. Our trip to the ICU would be detoured through the CT scan room. Andy was given a few milligrams of morphine intravenously and he became calmer, his blood pressure lower. Prior to leaving the ER, I asked the clerk to check with social service about finding a sign-language interpreter.

The scan confirmed my suspicion: the brain was covered with a white frosting around the cerebellum and occipital lobes—subarachnoid blood. The location of the bleeding pointed to an aneurysm on one of the arteries at the rear of the brain, the so-called posterior circulation. Such aneurysms are particularly dangerous to treat.

After the scan, Andy was taken to the ICU and the usual monitoring devices were inserted. He was given medications for sedation, blood pressure control, and seizure prevention, as well as some steroids to reduce brain swelling and inflammation. His parents still hadn't arrived and the hospital had not yet located an interpreter. These situations made me feel like a veterinarian rendering large-animal care. We probed, scanned, and medicated Andy with no way to communicate with him.

Ethically and legally, we had the right—the obligation—to do so, but it still made me feel very uncomfortable. Andy was awake but refused to read the messages we wrote for him. I could only imagine the fear and confusion of this poor deaf man whom we had stripped of all control of his body.

I notified Gary and the on-call attending neurosurgeon, Dr. Filipiano, of Andy's arrival and condition. Both agreed that Andy should be tucked in for the night and an emergency angiogram be scheduled for the following morning. Once we knew where the aneurysm was, we could better plan our operative attack upon it.

As surgeons, we can do little for the brain injury that a severe aneurysmal hemorrhage can inflict. We can, however, remove the risk of further hemorrhaging by surgically "clipping" the aneurysm. By making a window in the skull and peering at the tangle of blood vessels beneath the brain with an operating microscope, we can dissect the aneurysm sac away from the surrounding blood clot and place a tiny spring-loaded clip across the aneurysm's neck, the point where it arises from the feeding brain artery. Once the neck is clipped, the trapped aneurysm is rendered harmless.

This is one of medicine's most dangerous interventions. The lifting of the brain away from the skull base or the delicate microdissection of the aneurysm sac can cause explosive hemorrhage leading to rapid death. Moreover, the aneurysm clip may slip and occlude the parent artery and not the aneurysm, leading to stroke and disability. The brain, bulging and swollen from the hemorrhage, may be quite difficult to elevate from the bony skull. If it is lifted too forcefully, it will be bruised.

Surgery clearly saves the lives of many aneurysm patients, but the timing of such surgery is controversial. Every minute the patient lies in a hospital bed with a "live" aneurysm is a minute inviting another hemorrhage. Consequently, some experts hold that surgery to clip it should be done immediately.

Other experts have argued just as strongly that surgery within the first few days of a hemorrhage carries an increased risk which more than offsets the risk of waiting. During the earliest days after SAH, the brain is too swollen to lift easily and the aneurysm is very fragile to handle. Worse yet, the brain's arteries are angry and prone to even further spasm when exposed to the air. (You are never the same . . .) Early aneurysm surgery often means doing it at 3 A.M., when neither the surgeons nor the OR team are up to the task.

A compromise has been reached: early clipping of a ruptured aneurysm should be done only in patients with mild hemorrhages who look and feel relatively well after their initial headache. Andy was not in this group.

Andy's parents arrived later that evening. They looked to be in their early eighties and, though weathered, nimble and fit enough. Their clothes were rumpled from a long drive made even longer by the search for our hospital in an unfamiliar city. Like many large medical centers, our hospital sat in the middle of an urban university, a noisy and raucous neighborhood designed to confuse an elderly couple from a rural area.

I did my best to explain what had happened to Andy. SAH produces a minefield that the patient must navigate: rebleeding, vascular spasm, stroke, seizures, hydrocephalus, angiograms, major surgery. At any step something might explode, with the possibilities of paralysis, permanent nursing-home care, or death. I covered only the major issues that night, stopping short when Andy's mother began to become overwhelmed with all the bad scenarios. After having them sign a consent for his angiogram in the morning, I took them in to see their son.

Even though Andy was groggy from medication and his hands were loosely restrained to the bed, he began signing rapidly to his parents. They signed back. This interplay continued for several minutes as I stood outside the room.

I stepped up to the bed and asked them to introduce me to their son, which they did with a flurry of hand movements.

"Tell him he's going to be all right," I added. Another flurry. I used them as interpreters to explain to Andy about the upcoming angiogram.

After another fifteen minutes or so, Andy's nurse ushered them out, but before exiting, his father grasped Andy's hand and his mother kissed him. No doubt these displays of affection had sustained Andy through the numerous emotional traumas he must have endured in his life.

"Holy shit!" Gary expressed his usual hyperbolic amazement at the angiogram pictures. We sat drinking coffee on the morning following Andy's admission and reviewed the pictures as they came out of the X-ray processor. Andy was still on the angiogram table.

"He's got only a single vert!" Gary continued. The brain is normally supplied by four large arteries going through the neck: two carotid arteries in the front of the neck (the pulse that TV detectives search for before announcing that the victim is dead) and two vertebral arteries, "verts" in resident slang, running along the cervical spine in the back of the neck. Andy had only a single left vertebral artery. There was no sign of either a left or a right carotid artery or of the right vert—a bizarre congenital anomaly.

Gary puffed a cigarette and sipped his coffee. "Not only does he have just one vert, but it's got three aneurysms on it." He pointed out the three blebs with his smouldering cigarette tip. After the lone vertebral artery exited the neck and entered the base of Andy's skull, it branched out to supply the entire brain. Three aneurysm sacs, each about one-half inch in diameter, dangled like grapes from the branches.

Gary looked at me and smiled. "You know, Frank, it reminds me of that story about the obstetrician who goes to the new fathers' waiting room and says 'Mr. Johnson, I regret to tell you that your wife has just given birth to a ten-pound eyeball,' and the guys starts blubbering and says, 'Oh Jesus Christ, Doctor, what could be worse, what could be worse?!' The doctor puts his hand on the dad's shoulder and says, 'It's blind.' " Gary dragged on his cigarette again. "Well, Andy, you have only one artery in your entire fucking head. What could be worse? It has three aneurysms on it!"

The longer we worked together, the more I realized that Gary and I were kindred spirits. We were both of Slovak descent and from the blue-collar communities surrounding Pittsburgh. This background made us cruder, more blunt and much more prone to foot-in-mouth disease than the typical neurosurgical resident.

Gary was particularly good at getting into trouble with his mouth. One time in the surgeons' dressing room he repeatedly referred to one of our staff surgeons as "the stone-handed asshole" without realizing that the object of his tirade was just five feet away, relieving himself in one of the toilet stalls. Ever since that episode, Gary would admonish the residents to "check the crapper" before launching into any personal assaults. On some long nights on call, we still had deep discussions about the caliber of the stool if one is defecating and being insulted at the same time.

As a medical student, I often wondered why such incidents didn't get Gary canned. As I progressed in the program, I learned that it was because he was so good. Gary was the best technician our program had produced, a sort of surgical savant. Like people who can sit at the piano and play almost immediately, Gary mastered the most difficult operations so quickly that as chief resident he could run his operating room virtually unassisted. This enabled a staff surgeon to run two rooms at the same time, thus making twice as much money. The ability to generate staff-level billings on a paltry resident's salary gave Gary virtual immunity from punishments for his verbal adventures.

"What would you do with this character, Gary?" I asked.

"Me? I'd give him bigger doses of blood pressure meds, keep him in bed for about six weeks, and tell him to go home. You don't know which aneurysm has blown, so we'll have to clip all three. If you're jacking around with the wrong one and the bad one blows, kiss his ass goodbye. You can't place a temporary clip on his vert; it's the only pipe to his entire gourd. Too risky. I think trapeze artists call it 'working without a net.' Remember the rule: You can always make someone worse."

A temporary clip is used to clamp off the aneurysm's parent artery if the aneurysm starts bleeding again during surgery. This stops the bleeding so that the surgeon is not trying to deal with the aneurysm through a river of blood. Since most people have four brain arteries, clipping one of them for a few minutes is usually harmless. But Andy had no alternative routes for blood to get to his brain. Clipping his lone vertebral artery, even for a few seconds, might be lethal.

"So we don't do him?" I asked.

"I said if it was me, I wouldn't. It's not me, it's Filipiano, remember? He's aggressive. I bet he goes after these things. Real soon." Gary unfolded the crowded OR schedule sheet that was the chief resident's bible. "Like tomorrow."

As usual, Gary was on target. Dr. Filipiano came in that afternoon and discussed the situation with Andy and his parents. His presentation made surgery sound like the rational option.

In fact, clipping an aneurysm is a statistical operation. It is entirely possible for an aneurysm to bleed once and then never be heard from again, even without surgery. The statistics show only that SAH patients are *more likely* to live if they have surgery. Surgery doesn't guarantee a better outcome.

To operate on a bunion relieves the pain that is disrupting someone's life. There is no consideration of the "risks" of living with a bunion. Statistical operations, on the other hand, relieve no symptoms; they are done purely to lessen the risk of a disease in the future. For example, a woman may have an abnormal mammogram in a breast which is causing her no discomfort at all. Statistics show she will live much longer if she has the cancerous lump removed, even though it isn't bothering her.

The major difficulty with statistical operations is that it is impossible to predict the future of any one patient. It seems obvious that removing a cancerous breast lump is the correct choice for a healthy forty-two-year-old woman, but how about an eighty-one-year-old woman with diabetes, kidney failure, and end-stage heart disease? She may die of her other illnesses long before her cancer spreads, or the operation itself may do her in. The trick is to balance the risks of surgery against the risks of doing nothing, on a case-by-case basis. In Andy's case, Gary believed that the surgical risk might be greater than the risk of our doing nothing at all.

The course of an illness when doctors don't interfere with it is called its *natural history*. Ironically, for many diseases (including SAH), medicine has been fiddling with them for as long as they have been recognized as diseases. We are, therefore, totally clueless about the natural history of those diseases, except for what sparse data we can glean from patients who escape our clutches, either because they are too sick or have stubbornly refused our care.

Given this lack of hard data, a surgeon is left to choose the option for each patient. If the surgeon is aggressive, then the patient will be steered toward surgery. Unlike the bunion patient, who alone knows how much it hurts and how much surgical risk she is willing to assume to alleviate her suffering, candidates for statistical surgery are completely at the surgeon's mercy. Only the surgeon can provide the arguments for or against a statistical operation. Of course, the final decision rests with the patient and family.

Dr. Filipiano spiced his pre-op talk with graphic images of "bombs" in Andy's head that could explode and kill him at any instant. When all the talking was done, the shaken parents looked at each other. After a pause, Andy's father spoke the universal abdication of all who are confused by medical technology.

"Do what you think is best."

Music to a surgeon's ears.

The next morning I assisted Gary as he opened Andy's skull in preparation for the assault on the three "bombs" in his head. Gary let me drill some skull holes and widen them into the needed bony window, using large rongeurs. Just as Tom Sawyer could dupe his friends into believing fence painting was enviable work, chief residents could convince junior residents that this callous-forming drudgery was actually surgery.

After the skull window was fashioned and the posterior brain, or cerebellum, was exposed, Gary wheeled in the giant Contraves microscope. Looking like a small crane, with two sets of binocular eyepieces attached to a long, counterweighted boom, the scope was completely draped with sterile plastic sheets. The transparent drapes permitted the surgeon to manipulate the scope controls without becoming contaminated.

The operating microscope was first used for neurosurgery in the 1960s. Modern microscopes, with their fiber-optic halogen light sources, precision balancing, and stereoscopic vision, allow the neurosurgeon a superb view into the depths of a human head. For aneurysm surgery, the microscope was indispensable.

"Let Dr. Filipiano know that the dura is open and we're going under the scope," Gary instructed the circulating nurse. This gave the staff surgeon the option to come in as the operation was progressing to its more crucial phases. I had little doubt that Filipiano would come at once. Gary would not do this operation alone.

Gary proceeded by lifting the cerebellum at the rear of the brain, using a thin gold retraction blade fixed to a snakelike metal arm which was, in turn, fixed to the base on the OR table. He then used the hand controls on the scope so that he could see into the wound as he advanced the retractor further under the cerebellum. I watched through the observer's eyepieces of the microscope while the scrub nurse followed Gary's progress on a wall-mounted video screen connected to a TV camera within the microscope. The delicate folds and arteries on the cerebellar surface were like the terrain of some surreal planet under the glare of a fiber-optic sun.

The cerebellar surface was stained a dirty brown from the blood of Andy's original hemorrhage. Gary moved the retractor blade to the floor of the skull, searching for the main trunk of the vertebral artery as it entered the skull from the neck. With deft moves, he used thin dissectors and delicate knife blades to cleave away the scar tissue that already had begun to form between the brain and the skull.

"Remember, Frank, when we were interviewing to go into neurosurgery? They would look at your medical school grades, your research projects, whether you were an honor student and shit like that? Well—give me a micropatty please—well, none of that was worth a squat. I mean, how can you tell if someone can do this by what grades they made? A guy could have fingers like sausages, but because he got an honors in neuroanatomy they think he can become a microsurgeon. It doesn't make sense."

Microneurosurgery is indeed difficult. The surgeon can't look directly into the wound, but instead looks into the microscope eyepieces. This makes microsurgery similar to operating via remote control. Moreover, the powerful magnification of the scope makes even the slightest hand tremor seem like spastic gyrations. I thought about the agarose droplets.

"Well," Gary continued, "if I were a program chairman, do you know the first thing I would do when interviewing a prospective resident? I'd get out that Operation game—you know, the one with all the plastic pieces you have to pick out of small holes in a cardboard patient using electric tweezers? If you touch the patient with the tweezers, his nose lights up and a buzzer goes *honnnk* and scares the shit out of you. That's right, I'd say 'Here you go, pal, get out the fucking funny bone. No, not the breadbasket or the wrenched ankle, those are easy. I want the funny bone.' If he gets a *honnnk* before he pulls out the funny bone, I'd say 'Great grades, now get out.' If he can get me the funny bone, I know he has the hands for this."

"Is that fair?" I argued. "I mean, making the poor creep's whole future rest on that one task? Don't you think nerves might play a factor?"

"Of course, and that's the point," he countered. "In fact, I want them to be nervous. Anyone can have steady hands if they're relaxed. It's the ones who are granite under pressure that make the greatest surgeons." Maggie, the gung-ho cardiac chief, had also told me that pressure was part of the deal. All chief residents must think alike.

Gary adjusted the retractor and slowly pulled the cerebellum further away from the skull. The thick, pulsating vert came into view, and with it the blue, angry dome of the first aneurysm. At six-power magnification, the vertebral looked more like a redwood than an artery.

"How nervous does that son of a bitch make *you*?" He turned to me and winked.

I saw Dr. Filipiano enter the scrub area and begin putting on his surgical mask. A small man with a gaunt physique and wire glasses, Filipiano, only in his midforties, had already established a reputation as a master of complicated aneurysm cases. Like many neurosurgeons specializing in these "commando" cases, he carried a reputation for indifference to the death and destruction he sometimes left in his wake.

He was, as Gary acidly put it, the "prototypical surgical psychopath"—someone who could render a patient quadriplegic in the morning, play golf in the afternoon, and spend the evening fretting about that terrible slice off the seventh tee. At the time this sounded like a terrible thing, but I soon learned that Filipiano was no different from any other experienced neurosurgeon in this regard. He couldn't mourn every bad result—not without going insane. He handled hopeless cases on a daily basis. After one especially grisly complication, I asked Filipiano if surgery ever got to him. He quoted an old Russian saying: "People who cry at funerals shouldn't become undertakers."

Filipiano swung open the OR door and began drying his freshly scrubbed hands. "How's it going, chief?"

"I have the first aneurysm partly exposed," Gary said softly without looking away from the scope.

Filipiano was hurriedly gowned and gloved. He then unceremoniously displaced me from the observer's seat, relegating me to a stool in the corner. I watched the rest of the operation on the monitor.

There was a quiet lull in the OR as Gary and Filipiano tediously dissected the aneurysm away from the surrounding skull and brain, twisting the dome to and fro in search of the neck that joined it to the vertebral. I became hypnotized by the dull whine of the suctions, the soft clicking of the microscope motors, the hum of the bipolar coagulator being turned on and off.

In low murmurs, the two surgeons muttered into their masks: ". . . No, cut here. . . . Can that take a temporary clip? . . . Stop that oozing, please. . . . Use a ball dissector for that, goddamn it. . . . Clean the tips of this thing. . . ." I drifted into a twilight world between wakefulness and sleep. With my back pressed against the cold tile wall, I hallucinated about getting out of the hospital for an hour or two that evening. Maybe I'd go to the Black Angus for a hamburger. Although banished from the real action in this case, I was the dutiful junior resident: gowned, sterile, and technically impotent, unwilling to leave the OR for fear of appearing uninterested in what was happening on the fuzzy video screen.

Suddenly, a burst of frantic activity aroused me. Filipiano barked for a larger suction and the nurse-anesthetist pushed her alarm button to summon her staff anesthesiologist to the room. I looked at the monitor. The wound had turned red; the vertebral was gone and the cerebellum was now bathed with pulsatile waves of blood. Gary had slipped and plunged the sharp point of an arachnoid knife into the aneurysm dome.

Gary placed his suction deep into the wound. "Shit, oh shit . . . ," he moaned. The feeble microsuction did nothing to clear the field as bright blood gurgled audibly from the cranial wound and ran in angulated streams over the drapes.

"Do you want us to take his blood pressure down?" asked the nurse-anesthetist. Lowering the blood pressure with medication sometimes slowed the bleeding.

"No!" Filipiano responded sternly. "We need to temporary-clip and he'll need his blood pressure up. Just hang some blood, hang it now."

Working awkwardly from the assistant's chair, Filipiano jammed a giant glass-tipped suction into the wound and instantly the clear tubing filled with Andy's blood. On the monitor, I could see the large suction diverting the spewing column of blood sufficiently to see the vertebral artery once again. Gary remained frozen in the surgeon's chair, still clutching the useless microsuction.

"Give me a fifteen-millimeter straight temporary clip right away, now." Filipiano reached out with his right hand without looking away from the scope's eyepieces. The scrub nurse placed a long forceps bearing the open clip into his hand and gently guided it into the microscope's field of view. He swiftly placed the clip blades around the vessel and squeezed the clip shut. As dramatically as it had begun, the bleeding stopped. The staff surgeon quickly motioned for Gary to vacate the operator's chair.

"Call me the time, in minutes," Filipiano said to the anesthesiologist, who had just entered the room, "and load with barbiturates." The blood flow to Andy's brain was now ceased. The clock was running on his life. Filipiano had but a few minutes to repair the hole Gary had torn in the aneurysm's dome, or Andy would die. The barbiturates would protect Andy's brain somewhat, perhaps give them an extra few minutes.

The surgeon swiftly suctioned away the thick, fresh clot from around the now-collapsed aneurysm sac.

"One minute of clip time."

Working with reckless desperation, Filipiano tugged and pulled at the sac, peeling it away from the remaining adhesions. He was doing in seconds what would take thirty minutes or longer under more controlled conditions. Such vigorous tugging on the aneurysm ran the risk of ripping it completely away from the vertebral artery, leaving a gaping hole that could not be repaired. Finally, he was able to see the aneurysm's neck, where he could place a clip without obliterating the vertebral artery itself.

"Two minutes."

"Fifteen-millimeter bayonetted Yasargil clip."

The nurse handed him the long forceps again. He glanced at the clip and threw it back to her. "That's a temporary clip!" he cried shrilly, "don't kill this man, give me a permanent clip!" Temporary clips, because they are made to be placed on arteries and not on aneurysms, exert less force and cannot be expected to hold an aneurysm permanently closed. The nurse, in her haste, had loaded the wrong clip, wasting precious time.

"Three minutes."

The nurse rummaged frantically in the large gray tray of aneurysm clips, her hands quaking as she tried to load the requested clip onto the application forceps.

"Clip, clip, clip!" he screamed.

Filipiano finally seized the forceps and clip from her hands and loaded the clip himself. He thrust the clip's silver blades around the dome as it fluttered in the wake of air and frothy blood rushing up the adjacent suction tip. Slowly, he closed the blades down, killing the aneurysm.

"Four minutes. He's getting bradycardic." Andy's heart rate was falling; his brain was on the brink of oxygen starvation.

"Give me an empty clip applier." Filipiano removed the temporary clip from around the vertebral and the large vessel billowed once again with incoming blood. The clip on the aneurysm held. The bleeding did not return.

Filipiano decided to abandon the search for the remaining two aneurysms. He did not think Andy could tolerate another temporary occlusion of his vertebral artery, and he was convinced that the one he had just clipped was the aneurysm responsible for Andy's hemorrhage. He packed some soft gelatin foam around the clip and stepped out of the surgeon's chair, pulling off his gloves. "Close it up."

Gary sat motionless for a few minutes, his face pale. After Filipiano had left the room, I moved from my hiding place in the corner and walked up behind the sullen chief resident.

"Hey, Gary," I said over his shoulder.

"What?"

"Honnnnk."

He stared at me icily. "Fuck you."

* * *

We closed Andy's wound and wheeled him to the recovery room. Even after his anesthetic wore off, he remained unconscious and immobile from the large amount of barbiturates he had been given intraoperatively.

Gary sat at the nurses' station and began writing post-op orders. "If this guy wakes up from this fiasco," he whispered to me as he wiped his nose with his surgeon's cap, "I will go and take a dump on Center Avenue in broad daylight. How could his brain have survived five minutes of complete ischemia? Did you see how much back-bleeding there was from that vertebral? Zero."

I tended to agree with Gary. Five minutes of ischemia, or no blood flow, is usually a devastating insult to the nervous system. However, the effects of ischemia are difficult to predict. Andy was likely to have had some damage, some form of stroke, but where? And how bad would it be? Gary was betting that the damage was so profound as to render Andy forever comatose.

Filipiano told Andy's family that their son was likely to recover. He believed the episode of bleeding and ischemia was not long enough to cause irreversible injury. Filipiano was the eternal optimist.

We could only wait until the barbiturates wore off, two or three days.

On Thursday morning I met Gary at the door to the neurosurgical intensive-care unit for our usual 5:30 A.M. rounds. I escorted him down the hall to Andy's room.

"I've got something to show you." We went into the room, where Andy lay motionless, his belly bulging and his eyes closed. He still had a tracheal breathing tube and had not stirred a muscle since his Monday surgery.

"So?" Gary was impassive as he flipped through his index cards of patient data.

I vigorously rubbed Andy's chest with my knuckles, which prompted Andy to open his eyes and grab at my arm. The chief resident was startled. "Jesus Christ, the poor bastard's awake."

"That's right," I said, flashing a grin. I pulled a large wad of toilet paper from my white lab jacket and handed it to Gary. "Center Avenue's ten floors down, but you have to wait an hour or two, since it isn't broad daylight yet."

Except for some drooping of his left facial muscles, Andy appeared to have no paralysis. Later that afternoon, when his parents arrived, he even tried to communicate with them in sign language. On evening rounds, Filipiano pronounced the operation a success, hugged the parents, and gave the resident staff a heady discourse on how no blood flow is sometimes better than a little blood flow. Allowing some oxygen to the brain during a period of low blood flow permits the formation of destructive "free radicals," which does not occur if the blood flow is totally halted.

Over the ensuing days, however, Filipiano's beautiful free-radical theory was to be spoiled by an ugly fact: we couldn't wean Andy from the mechanical ventilator. Something was definitely wrong. The operation wasn't a complete success just yet. Each day Andy became brighter and more alert, passing us notes asking us to remove his breathing tube and allow him to eat. Every time we reduced the ventilator rate, however, he would start to hypoventilate and become lethargic, forcing us to restart the machine. When stimulated by being pinched he would breathe on his own for a brief time, only to stop breathing again when the stimulus ceased.

By the following week we had to insert a tracheostomy into his neck to avoid the complications of a long-standing endotracheal tube. We tried a variety of medications to make him breathe independently of his machine, including amphetamines, but nothing worked. As long as Andy was stimulated to breathe he would do so, but once his attention wandered, or if he started to fall asleep, he simply quit breathing. Tethered to a ventilator, Andy could not leave the intensive care unit.

Filipiano consulted Dr. Leo, one of the university neurologists. Dr. Leo's diagnosis: Ondine's curse.

We caught up with Dr. Leo in the cafeteria and asked him for further information regarding this rare condition.

"Ondine's curse," explained Dr. Leo as he peered over his half-glasses, "is a result of a stroke in the medulla, in the lower stem. That's where the respiratory drive center is located. As you know, we can either breathe voluntarily"—he demonstrated by taking a deep breath—"or involuntarily, without having to think about it. If our respiratory center is damaged, we can't breathe automatically; we have to think about each breath. Stop thinking about breathing, and we stop breathing. It's that simple."

"Who was Ondine? Some Queen Square neurologist?" asked Eric referring to the birthplace of neurology in London.

"No," laughed Dr. Leo, "Ondine was a nymph of

Greek mythology who offended the gods. As punishment, she was sentenced by Zeus to think about every breath. She knew she could never sleep, for to sleep meant death. That's a great curse, right?"

"Does it get better?" I asked.

"Not really, at least nowhere in the neurology literature. No, I think your friend had better give his ventilator a name. They will be companions for life."

Dr. Leo's observation was prophetic. A month passed after Andy's surgery, then two months, then three. Andy remained wedded to his ventilator. He could stay off it thirty minutes, just long enough to be wheeled to an outside courtyard for a respite from the intensive care unit. Andy had visitors during the first few weeks after surgery: the parish priest and some longtime members of the church's congregation. They never had much to say to him, but then they probably never had much to say to him when he was well, either. As Andy languished in the hospital for months, his parents were the only people who continued to come.

An ICU is a terrible place to live, a place of no night and no day, just eternal light. Ventilator alarms sound at all hours, night-shift personnel laugh and swap stories, cleaning people roam at all hours. The private tasks of life, like bathing or having a bowel movement, are afforded little privacy. The disorienting effect of the ICU environment can cause psychosis in otherwise normal individuals. Andy's deafness was probably a blessing in the ICU world. It gave him some peace.

At the time, our hospital had no protocol for managing ventilator-dependent patients outside of an ICU. The rising costs of hospital care would eventually force hospitals to deal with ventilators on regular wards, nursing homes, and even in private homes, but those developments were still a decade away. His years of smoking and chronic pneumonias would have made it difficult for him to leave the ICU for more than a week or two anyway, even if his ventilator were moved to a regular hospital bed.

The ICU became Andy's home. He dressed in street clothes and tennis shoes and watched television in an easy chair, his ventilator hoses draped across his belly. A large crucifix was hung on the back wall, beside a get-well message from the diocesan bishop.

Four months passed. We pushed the limit of medical technology to help him. A portable, vacuum-driven clamshell respirator was fitted to his body, a modern version of the old iron lung. Andy's round body did not take well to the machine and it never worked properly.

Andy grew more and more despondent. He became inseparable from his rosary and prayed constantly. One day in early December, the fifth month of his hospitalization, I was summoned to the ICU because Andy was having an outburst. For no apparent reason, he had become violent, crying hysterically. He had overturned his bedside stand and hurled his rosary at one of the nurses.

I wrote him a note, asking him what was wrong. He just shook his large head, made some hand signals, and waved me out of the room. We gave him an injection of the sedative Haldol and located his parents, who had become ICU fixtures themselves, in the hospital gift shop. After communicating with Andy for several minutes, they emerged from his room appearing shaken.

"What's wrong with him, Mrs. Wood? Is he having pain?"

Her eyes filled with tears and she pointed to a small Christmas tree which the nurses had just that morning set up in the corner of the ICU.

"He didn't know it was getting close to Christmas; he had lost track of time. He wants to leave here and decorate the church. We told him that he knows he cannot leave, and he said he wants to die."

"He's been very depressed . . . ," I started, but Andy's father stopped me.

"We know, son. We know you have done everything you could. But we think he's right." He stopped and gained his composure. "We want him to die, too."

Andy eventually calmed down, but he remained sullen and bitter. Christmas came and went. A psychiatrist was consulted and prescribed some antidepressant medications, which helped little. The residents learned a rudimentary sign language, but Andy ignored anyone except his parents.

The left-sided facial paralysis he had suffered during surgery had never fully resolved, but it was not much of a problem until late January, when his left eye turned red and swollen. Because of the paralysis, Andy could not fully close the left eye. He had suffered repeated abrasions to his cornea over the past months, but they had all healed quickly before. This time, though, the cornea became infected and, despite antibiotics, developed scar tissue. His other eye was already blind; now the corneal scarring clouded his remaining vision. By February, Andy was totally blind.

This pushed him over the edge. He began pulling out his tracheostomy and pushing the ventilator out of the room. Soon he had to be continuously tied to the bed and sedated to prevent him from committing suicide. His parents tried making signs against his chest and hands to get him to understand them, but he either couldn't or wouldn't sign back. Whenever the hand restraints were removed for him to write a note, he immediately grabbed for the tracheostomy, trying to break the one restraint that bound him to the living. One day on rounds, Gary and I stood and watched as Andy grimaced and strained against the leather restraints while the ventilator pumped unwanted air into his lungs.

"I think it was Wyatt Earp who said 'Any day above ground is a good day,' " mused Gary, "but Wyatt never met this guy."

In late February, Andy's parents called a conference with Dr. Filipiano. They requested that Andy's ventilator be turned off. The case was taken to the hospital's ethics committee, which was nervous about approving this. Andy no longer spoke for himself; how could the committee be sure he wanted to die? The parents asked the ethics committee to come and see Andy, imprisoned in a bed, blind, deaf, ventilated against his will, his lungs wracked with pneumonia. The committee obliged and made a trip to the ICU. Shortly thereafter, they approved the request.

At 11:00 P.M. on the evening after the request was granted, Gary and I met the Woods in the ICU. Andy's mother kissed him on the forehead and then began tracing something into his hands with her index finger.

Andy nodded vigorously. A respiratory technician disabled the ventilator alarm with her key. Gary and I stood looking at each other, wondering who would pull the tracheostomy and be the executioner du jour. Before either of us could act, however, Andy's father motioned for everyone to leave the room. He then closed the door and pulled the window curtains shut.

I waited for an hour or so but no one emerged from the room. I went to bed. At about four in the morning the ICU called me to pronounce Andy Wood dead. When I arrived, his mother and father were sitting on either side of his giant, lifeless body, still holding his hands, alpha and omega—present at the beginning, present at the end.

His mother stared serenely at her only child through her reddened eyes. There is an old curse: "May you outlive all of your children." Mrs. Wood now lived this nightmare. She looked up at me and spoke. "They said to put him in a home when he was just a child, but we couldn't do that. Now, we were afraid he'd end up in a nursing home. We couldn't do that, either. He had a good life. He was a good son . . ."

Her voice trailed off. The jumbled chromosomes of decades past had turned out to be no mistake to her at all. By her face, I could tell that he would always be the most perfect little boy in the world.

The next morning, Gary and I rounded in the intensive care unit without making further reference to Andy. Gary must have known that his small slip with the arachnoid knife had been as deadly for Andy as a shotgun blast, but the chief resident never spoke about the case again.

Gary's metamorphosis into a surgical psychopath was now complete. I admired Gary, but he showed not the slightest remorse or concern for his lethal error. He had described Filipiano's surgical callousness with disdain; he now achieved it himself. Like me, he had entered the chrysalis of residency as the son of a steelworker, little more than a boy out of medical school. In four months he would emerge from his seven years of training with neurosurgeon's wings. Was this just an act? Was psychopathy part of this transformation? And, I wondered, would I follow his path to indifference? Would my compassion start to slip away?

Perhaps. But perhaps patients didn't want compassion from brain surgeons. They might prefer Nietzsche to Alan Alda, a superman who would make them better— even if he didn't give a shit. Unfortunately, Gary fulfilled neither role for Andy.

I would have to learn to quit crying at funerals.

8

If It Was Easy, Everyone Would Do It

My junior year of residency was near an end. On a Friday evening in May, Gary, Eric, and I finished rounds about eight o'clock and went to the surgeons' lounge to change into our street clothes. The intern was "in the house" that night and Gary, who was responsible for backing him up, was in no hurry to head home. An intern can make very few decisions on a specialty service such as neurosurgery, and, as chief resident, Gary never strayed far from the hospital on the nights that the intern took call.

"Who wants some Roma's pizza?" he shouted down the long row of lockers. Roma's pizza parlor was directly across the street from the hospital. So many of the residents ate at Roma's that a direct hospital line had been installed there.

"No thanks," Eric replied. He had been on call the night before and was anxious to see his wife and children. Eric was dedicated to his work but made a quick exit when the work was done. I never liked to hang around the hospital campus and socialize either, but I decided to go because I hated to see the chief eat alone— even if it meant inhaling his cigarette smoke and bullshit another two hours.

"I'll go, if you buy," I agreed.

"It's a deal," said Gary, "but you have to obey Gary's law of eating pizza."

"Another law?! What's this one?"

"You'll just have to wait and see."

We hurried through the hospital lobby, casting quick glances around corners and down hallways to be sure that we didn't accidentally bump into any attending surgeons or patient families who might want to discuss business. A chief resident never finishes a workday, he just sort of amputates it. There was always something more to do if he looked too hard. This night, all was quiet. We made our escape undisturbed.

Roma's was filled with the usual crowd of residents. Every specialty was represented, each identifiable by a characteristic uniform and behavior. Two bulked-up orthopedic residents were taking a break from their anobolic steroids and downing a few calzones instead. A general surgery resident, still dressed in surgical scrubs and wearing blood-splattered shoe covers, was slamming his hips into a "Star Wars" pinball machine and cursing.

In the back corner of the pizza parlor a table was crammed with medical residents dithering about some liver syndrome, their stethoscopes draped around their necks and their coat pockets jammed with standard-issue medical resident paraphernalia: the Washington Manual, index cards, photocopies of *New England Journal* articles, syringes. The pediatric residents were essentially medical residents with small teddy bears wrapped about their pastel-colored stethoscopes and an empathetic gaze permanently welded onto their faces.

As we passed the table of medical residents, Gary glanced back at me and began scratching violently at the back of his right ear with his cupped hand, imitating a dog scratching a flea. This was his own personal code for internists. In resident lexicon, internal medicine residents are "fleas." The origin of this epithet is unknown, although several colorful theories have been advanced: fat, loud, egotistical assholes; the last creatures to jump on a dying dog.

There is a constant tension between internists and surgeons, the internists viewing surgeons as brainless technicians, the surgeons viewing internists as medical Neros fiddling as patients burn. This internecine feud peaks during residency and eases after a few years in practice. New surgeons soon realize that their patients, and mortgage payments, depend upon internists. Internists soon realize a surgeon isn't such a bad person to have around when a patient is vomiting blood.

Gary and I ordered a large pizza and found an open booth. The chief lit a cigarette. "Look at those goddamn fleas, jabbering about some disease they'll see once in their lifetimes. That's the trouble with fleas, they only like the bizarre stuff. They hate their bread-and-butter cases. That's the difference between us and the fucking fleas. See, we love big juicy lumbar disc herniations, but they hate hypertension. The pediatric fleas—maybe we should call them gnats?—hate healthy babies. They dream about seeing some poor kid with cystic fibrosis. When we see a guy with pain shooting down his leg, we don't cross our fingers and hope he's got a signet cell cancer growing into his parasympathetic plexus like they do. We hope he's got some garden-variety disc rupture that we can fix and then kiss his ass goodbye."

He paused to puff his shortening cigarette and quickly changed the subject. "What staff guy is on call this weekend?"

"Fred," I answered, expecting the chief's reaction.

"Oh, fuck," Gary grimaced. "I hope nothing comes in this weekend. I have a month to go and if I can get out of this place without doing another case for that dick-with-ears I'll be a happy man."

"He's a big fan of yours, too, pal, ever since the bone flap thing." The bone flap incident had occurred early in Gary's chief year. Fred and Gary were performing a cranial operation to remove a benign brain tumor. Fred had performed the entire operation himself—a grave insult to a chief resident, known as "stealing the case." After Fred left the OR, further irritating the chief by dumping upon him the tedium of closing the wound, an angry Gary had engraved the phrase "Fred sucks" with the electrocautery knife on the inside of the bone flap, the plate of skull bone that is temporarily sawed away to gain access to the brain. He had then wired the flap back into place, thinking that the inside of the patient's skull would never again see the light of day.

Unfortunately, the bone flap developed a staph infection and had to be removed a week later. Once contaminated with bacteria, the free piece of skull must be removed to cure the infection. The soft spot is filled in with plastic several months later. Gary coerced me into assisting Fred with the surgical removal of the infected flap. I'll never forget the almost unintelligible stream of invectives that spewed forth when Fred saw Gary's skull graffiti. Fred was too embarrassed to send the discarded flap to the pathology department as it was, and we spent an hour drilling the message off the bone before allowing it to leave the OR.

"Screw him." Gary was characteristically unrepentant. "It was a tiny convexity meningioma and he stole the whole thing. How should I know the flap would get infected?"

"Well, you should be happy he didn't tell the administration about it," I said, trying to maintain some fairness.

"Are they going to fire me for one skull-o-gram? Where's that pizza? You were a physics major, weren't you, Frank? You know about quantum states? Well, I have two quantum states: hungry and nauseated. It's a curse. I have to eat until I'm nauseated, or I stay hungry." Gary had the lanky, wiry build of the chain-smoking, eat-anything-and-everything-and-never-gain-a-pound, type A personality. He could consume vast quantities of food.

The waitress delivered the pizza several minutes later.

"And now," I asked, "what's Gary's law of pizza-eating?"

Gary pulled the pizza toward him and removed half of it, folding it in two and biting into it like a giant sandwich.

"When I share a pizza with someone," he replied with a full mouth, "it's not fifty-fifty—it's whoever eats the fastest gets the most. That's Gary's law. So you better get started."

I was no match for him. I managed to eat only two of the eight slices before Gary had devoured the rest. When we were finished, the chief leaned back in the booth and closed his eyes contentedly.

"Nauseated?" I asked. He gave a slight smile and nodded. I probed him about his future plans. "Have you decided what job you're going to take?"

Gary was silent for a few minutes, as if he was drifting off to sleep. He then opened his eyes and bolted forward, reaching for his nearly empty pack of cigarettes.

"I took that job in upstate New York. You know, the

old fart who says he wants to retire in two years and turn his one-million-a-year practice over to me."

"Really?" I was amazed. "You interviewed for that job five months ago. When did you decide to go there?"

"Five months ago. I signed a contract when I was there."

"But you've interviewed at a dozen places since then! Why didn't you tell anyone you were already taken?"

Gary laughed, blowing pulses of smoke. "Naive boy," he whispered, leaning close, "if you're a good candidate, people will fly you anywhere to interview. And each interview gets you out of this meat grinder for a day or two. Why the fuck would I tell people I signed a contract five months ago and quit interviewing? Look at where I've been since: San Diego, San Francisco, New York—shitty jobs every one of them, but great trips. I didn't go to Akron, did I? You see, that's the job of the chief resident, Frank. Everyone thinks we're here to teach you punks how to sew and tie, but you can learn that shit anywhere. We're here to teach you really important things, like how to con a dinner at Antoine's out of a private-practice group in New Orleans that you wouldn't work for if your life depended on it."

I was a Buddhist pupil seated in the presence of the Enlightened Master.

"The next five years of your life, Frank, will be hard," Gary continued, "but always remember this: If neurosurgery wasn't hard, everyone would do it. Look at those fleas over there. Do you think they really *want* to write prescriptions for Inderal for the next forty years? Do you think they wake up at night screaming 'Dialysis! I must dialyze one more patient!' Maybe a few do, but most of them wanted to be surgeons but just couldn't hack the work it takes to be one. If a genie popped out of their pizza right now and said he could make them into any type of doctor they would want to be, right here and now, which one of them do you think would say 'Oh, genie please make me a gastroenterologist so that I could look up someone's ass all day and my office can be filled with spastic-colon patients wanting to show me Polaroids of their latest bowel movement,' or 'Genie, I get an erection just thinking about chronic lung patients coughing up goobers at me.' No way. They'd all want to be heart surgeons or brain surgeons or transplant surgeons."

Gary's beeper went off. It was the emergency room. He dunked his last cigarette into his cup of flat Coke with a hiss and headed for the hospital phone. I watched as he stood hunched over with a finger in his other ear to block out the incessant noise from the video games. He listened for a few minutes, nodded his head, and hung up. He returned to the booth, threw a ten-dollar bill on the table, and grabbed his jacket without sitting down. "Let's go."

"Go where?" I asked, bewildered. "I'm not on call."

"Do you want to learn how to be a neurosurgeon or are you going to go home and watch *Gilligan's Island*? You can tell some future patient that you had to skip learning about spine trauma because you just had to see the episode where Mr. Howell decides to put Skipper in his will."

"All right, all right, I'm coming, but I have to call Kathy first. She's expecting me." My future wife was growing used to my last-minute cancellations.

"Call her from the ER. Walter has some guy who rolled his pickup truck and is getting weak in front of his eyes. You know Walter, he wants to be a plastic surgeon. Stuff like this just panics the shit out of him." Walter was our intern. He was a good intern, but definitely more of a Bel Air boob-lifter than an urban trauma surgeon.

As we were on our way out, one of the orthopedic residents called to us. "Hey, Gary, going back again? Don't you guys ever leave?"

"Man, this is a tough year for us, Bob," Gary retorted, "but nothing like those three toughest years in an orthopedic surgeon's life."

"Yeah, what are those?"

"Second grade." We exited into the dark street and headed for the ER entrance.

The ER looked a lot like Roma's: brightly lit, filled with residents, and humming with electronic beeps and whistles. We tossed our jackets in the nursing station and went to the trauma room. Walter met us there, thin and handsome. An ugly plastic surgeon is about as successful as a fat aerobics instructor. Walter was obviously relieved to see us. Most interns enter our program knowing less neurosurgery than the housekeeping people. When on our service, they wander about clumsily, literally living out the nightmare of being on stage without knowing a single line of the play.

"Walt, my man." Gary put his arm around the frazzled intern. "What have you got for us here?"

Walt pulled out his crib sheet filled with random pencil marks. "Billy Renaldo, age thirty-three, no prior medical history, was coming home from softball practice when his pickup truck was sideswiped as he came off a ramp onto Route 8 . . . his truck flipped over . . . Uh, let's see . . . his vitals at the scene were—"

"Wait," said Gary, "do I look like I'm from Haaah-vard? Just the facts. Is he alive, is he awake, does he move anything? Is he really thirty-three and still called 'Billy'?"

The intern didn't miss a beat. "He never lost consciousness. He came in about half an hour ago saying that his neck hurt and that his legs felt heavy, but he could move them OK. But now he says he can't move them at all and his hands are feeling 'tingly.' He has no external marks of trauma and the general surgeons are done with him. He really looks pretty good."

Gary didn't wait to hear more. He darted into the trauma room. The patient, a tanned, muscular man with a shock of black hair and a black mustache, was strapped to a backboard and still wearing his softball uniform.

"Mr. Renaldo," Gary began, "I'm Dr. Stancik, chief resident in neurosurgery, and this is Dr. Vertosick and Dr. Schwartz." He motioned to Walter and me. "Try and wiggle your toes."

"Call me Billy. And I can't. I could about ten minutes ago, and now they just won't do it."

"Move anything from the hips down."

Billy weakly rotated his legs at the hips.

"Try lifting them," Gary instructed as he loosened the restraining belts holding Billy to the backboard. No luck.

"Doc," Billy continued, "now my hands feel funny. Jesus Christ, what's happening to me?"

"Don't panic," said Gary sternly, "we'll figure it out." The chief examined the distraught man completely and then we left the room while some spine X rays were taken.

"He's got a C7 sensory-level," Gary whispered to me, "and a nearly complete motor-level as well. He looks good, all right, except he's paraplegic. Walter's idea of 'good' needs some revision." C7 referred to the seventh cervical vertebra, at the junction of the neck and chest. Billy's spinal cord wasn't working below that level, giving him numbness and paralysis from about his armpits down. Gary thought out loud: "But why is he progressing so quickly? He was moving his legs when he came in."

"Maybe he wasn't properly immobilized," I offered. If his neck was broken, improper movements could injure the spinal cord further.

"Naw," said Gary, "he looks pretty immobilized to me and, besides, he's wide awake. If someone breaks his neck and is wide awake, they're in so much pain you could lift them up by their nostrils and they wouldn't move their necks. Something fishy is going on here."

"Maybe he's having a conversion reaction," chimed an emergency medicine resident.

"Possible," mused Gary, "maybe he struck out in the bottom of the ninth and his male pride made him a paraplegic to save face . . . but don't call the psychiatrists in just yet."

The phrase "conversion reaction" is a euphemism for hysteria. The patient "converts" an emotional trauma, such as a failed marriage or, in Billy's case, the shock of being nearly killed in an accident, into a physical complaint such as blindness or the paralysis of an arm or a leg. Although the symptom has no organic cause, the patient isn't faking in the conventional sense, either. Malingerers don't *believe* that they are ill. That's why hidden cameras catch them throwing away their wheelchairs when they think no one is watching. The hysteric, on the other hand, is truly convinced that the illness is real, and will continue to manifest symptoms even when alone. A patient with hysterical numbness will let a needle be pushed through a fingertip without flinching.

The word "hysteria" derives from *hyster*, Greek for uterus and root word of "hysterectomy." Ancient physicians believed hysteria to be an exclusively female disease. While it remains more common in women, I had seen plenty of conversion reactions in men, too. In fact, anybody can turn hysteric, even people with no obvious mental-health problems.

The X rays were done. I reviewed them with Gary in a back room. The cervical and thoracic spine films showed no evidence of fractures or dislocation of vertebrae.

"See," the ER resident chided, "I told you, he's hysteric. Let's just watch him for a while. I'll bet you he walks out the door."

Gary squinted at the film for another few minutes and then wheeled about. "No . . . no, no, no. He has a sensory-level, ascending paralysis and neck pain. Frank, get on the horn to Fred, let him know what's going on. . . . Walter, call the radiology resident, tell him we need a C1 puncture for a myelogram and CT. And I mean now, as in now and not two hours from now. I'll call the OR and tell them we're coming up as soon as the myelogram is done."

A myelogram involves instilling some iodine dye directly into the fluid space around the spinal cord, followed by X rays and a CT scan to trace the flow of the dye down the spinal column. Gary wanted the dye injected at C1, just behind the ear.

"What do you expect to find?" I asked. "His films are normal."

"I don't know," Gary answered, "a disc rupture, a clot, maybe. But we have to look." In tense situations, Gary's flippant facade was jettisoned, exposing a tenacious and humorless professional beneath. He reminded me of the bomber pilot from the movie *Dr. Strangelove*, a buffoonish bumpkin until he receives his orders to deliver a hydrogen bomb on Moscow, at which time he is transformed into a fanatic and competent cold warrior.

We returned to the trauma room and Gary explained the myelogram test to Billy. As we were leaving to head upstairs to radiology, Billy called out: "Doc . . ."

Gary returned to the bedside. "Call me Gary."

"Gary," the man said quietly, "I can't move my fingers anymore."

The adult spinal cord is about two feet long and barely larger than the little finger in girth, passing down the middle of our backs encased in the bony armor of the vertebral column. Through this thin ribbon of fatty nervous tissue courses life. The spinal cord is notoriously intolerant of injury. Like IRS agents and Mafia dons, the cord will tolerate a certain level of insult, but wise men don't push to that level.

While portrayed as the "main nerve" connecting the brain to the rest of the body, the spinal cord is more than just a nerve. In fact, it is a complex organ possessing an intelligence of its own. Stereotyped movements, like standing and walking, are preprogrammed within the spinal cord's gray matter. This frees up our cerebrums to do those things which it does best, such as writing sonatas and inventing lite beer ad campaigns.

In lower animals, the cerebrum is so primitive that complicated motor behaviors originate in the spinal cord out of necessity. There just aren't enough neurons in puny nonprimate brains to accommodate the "software" necessary to power all of the fins, wings, and feet. A headless chicken can run about *sans* brains. Our neurophysiology department once made a few brainless cats for a vision experiment, later giving them away as pets to unsuspecting cat-lovers who couldn't tell them from intact animals. ("My Muffin is so smart . . . she knows her name, she is just too independent and finicky to come when I call her . . .")

As any athlete can verify, thinking too much during competition can hurt performance of repetitive tasks. The higher brain is always trying to embellish movements like a tennis forehand or golf drive, when such actions are best left to the spinal cord alone.

In humans, the "brainlike" behavior of the spinal cord can have macabre consequences. Patients with brains killed by gunshot wounds, hemorrhages, or other injuries can dupe family members, friends, even nurses, into believing that they are awake. An arm reaches up to grab a coat lapel, a hand grasps the hand of a loved one, a leg withdraws in apparent pain after a hospital tray is dropped on it—all preprogrammed spinal reflexes. Called "Lazarus movements" for obvious reasons, these reflexes make it difficult to convince a bereaved family that their loved one is, in fact, legally dead and should be removed from life support.

A spinal cord injury is either "complete" or "incomplete." A complete injury deprives the patient of all sensation and movement below the level of the injury. If the spinal cord is injured in the upper back, between the shoulder blades, the patient will have no movement in the legs, no bowel or bladder control, and no sensation below the nipples. A complete neck injury will produce paralysis involving the arms as well as the legs. When the injury occurs very high in the neck, near the base of the skull, the muscles of respiration will be paralyzed and the patient usually asphyxiates before help arrives. A successful hanging produces this injury.

If the patient displays any movement or sensation below the level of the injury, even the faint wiggle of a toe or a two-inch patch of feeling on the inner thigh, the injury is said to be incomplete. This is a crucial distinction. Complete spinal-cord injuries virtually never improve, while incomplete injuries, even severe ones, can reverse with time and proper treatment.

Gary and I walked up two flight of stairs to the X-ray department in silence. His head was down and his brow furrowed in thought. He was agonizing over what to do for Billy. Suddenly, he stopped and turned to me. "Forget the myelogram. Frank, go downstairs and get that guy to sign a consent for an exploratory laminectomy. I'm going up to the OR and make sure they're set up and an anesthesia resident is available."

"Why are we skipping the myelogram?"

"He's going downhill before our eyes; if we wait much longer he's going to stop breathing and the horse will be out of the barn. He can't have just ruptured a disc in his neck, because that shouldn't cause the weakness in his legs to ascend into his arms. He may be crazy, but I wouldn't bank on that, either. I've seen a lot of conversion reactions and none of them gets worse with time. He must have an epidural clot that's expanding. At least that's what I think." Gary turned and began running up the stairs, calling back to me in a feigned British accent: "Hurry, Watson, the game is afoot! Bring your revolver!"

The epidural space lies between the cardboardlike

covering of the brain and spinal cord, called dura, and the skull and vertebrae. It is a space densely packed with veins which can be torn during trauma. While epidural blood clots are common in the head, where they compress the brain and cause coma, they are distinctly uncommon in the spine. Gary was guessing. I bet he had never even *seen* a traumatic epidural in the spine before. If he was wrong, we could be subjecting a man suffering from transient hysteria to a risky and painful operation. If he was right, and we waited to get the myelogram to prove it, the spinal cord might be hopelessly damaged. Gary had decided that a hysteric with an incision was better than a quadriplegic with pretty myelogram films.

I returned to the ER. Billy's wife was sitting by the stretcher, holding his now limp hand and crying. I stopped short of entering the room.

"Where are the kids?" I overheard him ask.

"With my mom," she replied, "they're going to spend the night there."

"Good, good . . . I don't know how long I'll be here. My bank card isn't in my wallet, it's on the 'fridge . . ."

Life goes on. Honey, call the plumber and, by the way, I'm paralyzed. I broke in and introduced myself. I examined Billy again. He could no longer grasp with either hand and his biceps were weaker. He still had a few areas of sensation in his legs, although they remained paralyzed. Excellent, I thought, he's still incomplete.

I explained that the myelogram would take an hour or two to set up and complete and so we had decided to go ahead and take Billy to the OR and explore his spine. If we didn't do something soon, he might die from the advancing paralysis. After I was through talking, there was a pause. Billy took a deep breath and then spoke. "Let's do it. But give me a minute with my wife, alone."

I left the room and closed the door. I found Walter stretched across a tattered vinyl sofa in the ER lounge. "Give them five minutes," I instructed the intern, "and get him upstairs to the OR. Call Fred back and tell him where we are." There would be the expected spousal grief when it came time to take Billy upstairs, and I didn't want to be there. These pathetic scenes, like exposure to X rays, are occupational hazards that take a cumulative toll on a physician's health. I avoided them whenever I could. I wasn't a complete psychopath just yet.

I changed back into surgical scrubs and met Gary in operating room eight. Chun, a senior anesthesia resident, was setting up his machines and Lisa, our scrub tech, was opening a package of sterile instruments.

"We're on our own, buddy," Gary said through his mask. "Two other rooms are still running and there isn't any circulating nurse. Do-it-yourself neurosurgery. Help me with this." Gary yanked a large metal-and-Styrofoam contraption from the bottom of the OR cupboard. It was the laminectomy frame, used to hold patients prone on the operating table.

The circulating nurse assists with setting up the room. During an operation, the "circulator" serves as an all-purpose gofer, answering phones, opening suture material, checking pagers, and so on. When the OR was understaffed, as it usually was in the evenings and on weekends, circulating nurses were pressed into duty as scrub nurses.

Walter arrived minutes later, pushing Billy on his

stretcher. Just then the OR phone rang. Chun answered it, then handed the receiver to Gary. "It's for you." Gary thrust the frame at me and took the phone.

"Yeah . . . Oh, hello, Fred . . . yeah, he must have a clot . . . No, I didn't get any studies, but he's ascending . . . What? Uh-huh . . . of course I gave him steroids. . . . I'm going to start at about T3 and work up. . . . OK, we'll be here. See you later."

Gary hung up, his eyes narrowing above his mask. "A dick-with-ears, that's what he is. He's pissed because we have no myelogram, but he's going to have to stay pissed. He only wants a myelogram because he's at the symphony and it would have delayed the case until after he's heard his fucking Beethoven. He'll show up two hours late, anyway. Let's get started." He then called out to Walter, who was standing in his street clothes outside the OR, baby-sitting Billy. "Get dressed, amigo, we need you to circulate in here."

Gary and I wheeled the stretcher into the small OR, parking it parallel to the OR table. The patient would be anesthetized on the stretcher and then flipped onto his stomach on the OR table after he was asleep. Gary examined him again. Billy's large biceps muscles were now both totally flaccid. "Relax, ace, Dr. Chun here is going to put you to sleep. See you soon." We then sat on stools in the corner and let Chun do his work.

The room was quiet. Contrary to popular belief, operating rooms are not always crowded, dramatic, and noisy. Nor are there choirs of seraphim basking in the glow of a larger-than-life surgeon. The OR can be an insufferably intimate place, an arena where an intensely personal transaction occurs: the bartering of one person's skill for another's quality of life. There we gathered, two men from a pizza shop, one man from a softball diamond, and an anesthesiologist, spending a tragic Friday evening together.

Chun glided an endotracheal tube into Billy's throat and began taping it to the sleeping man's face. I swiftly placed a bladder catheter into Billy and then the three of us, Gary, Chun, and I, grunted and heaved Billy over onto the Wilson frame and positioned him to our satisfaction. "Shit," said Gary as he stared down at Billy's broad, tanned back, now faceup on the OR table, "this guy's built like a rock. What a waste if we don't get his cord back."

After we had scrubbed and draped the operative area, Gary and I took our positions on opposite sides of the table. "Knife," Gary said softly. Lisa suspended the Bard-Parker blade between us, but Gary didn't move to take it. He just stood and looked at me. "Well, are you going to take it or not? I didn't tear you away from the Skipper and his little buddy just to watch me do a case, did I?"

"Me?"

"You'll be a senior resident before you know it. C'mon, bring this guy's legs back to life for him."

I took the knife. Gary placed his right index finger on the nape of Billy's neck and his left index finger in the middle of his back, just below the rib cage. "Between here and here . . . let's go, don't be shy." I slid the knife on a line between Gary's hands and took the incision deep through the skin and fatty tissues. The incision was over a foot and a half in length. "Now get your hot knife," Gary continued to instruct me. I grabbed the electrocautery pen and began carving the thick meat of Billy's back from the spinal bones below. Gary swept away the tissue with large silver scoops as I detached it with the heat. This allows access to the spine, but does no permanent damage since muscle can heal.

About ninety minutes later, we had exposed the laminae of the spine from the neck down to the midback. The laminae are bony shingles which extend along the length of the spine and protect the back of the spinal cord. "OK," said Gary as he probed under the edge of one of the laminar shingles with a small curette, "get a Kerrison punch under here and get to work." The Kerrison is a long-handled metal tool with a small biting cup at the tip. It's used to chip small pieces of bone away, bit by bit. Removing the thick protective bone in this manner is tedious, but it is the only safe way given the delicate organ below. Removing the laminae, a procedure known as laminectomy, is like chiseling through a cinder block to reach an egg encased within—without cracking the shell.

We removed one lamina, at the fourth thoracic level, and found nothing but pristine dura. No clot. I could almost feel Gary's stomach churning with a mixture of doubt and pepperoni. "Keep going," he barked, "it's got to be here. Look, the dura isn't pulsating." The lack of pulsations was evidence, albeit weak, that some compression of the cord existed above our laminectomy.

I kept chipping away. Piece by piece, the third thoracic lamina ended up in the silver pan on Lisa's Mayo stand. Still no clot. "I think the dura is pulsating here," I observed, trying to be scholarly. Gary was unimpressed. "Keep going, tiger. Higher."

In and out of the cavernous wound I went, dipping my tiring hand down to the spinal canal, grasping a bite of bone, and then releasing it into a specimen pan. Grasping and releasing, grasping and releasing, in and out, in and out. A widening expanse of translucent dura, the spinal cord visible just below, grew at the depths of the red wound. I had never worked around the spinal cord before and my arms were tense as I painstakingly guided the metal rongeur repeatedly under the laminae. My fatigue was growing, but I could not show weakness. *If it was easy, anybody could to it.*

Suddenly, just below the cut edge of the second thoracic lamina, a small piece of clot, resembling fresh liver, peeked out around the left side of the spinal dura. "There!" Gary shouted with the enthusiasm of a prospector seeing the glint of gold in his pan. He grasped the Kerrison from my hand and began making swift, sure strokes, slicing through the lamina like a rower slicing through a river. The clot grew larger and larger as the spinal opening proceeded higher. "Oh, sorry," he apologized, handing the instrument back to me, "you're doing fine."

Hour after hour, I pulled bone away as Gary suctioned the thick epidural clot. Fred showed up, peered into the wound, and retreated to the lounge to sleep. At 5 A.M., over six hours into surgery, we reached the top of the clot at the fourth cervical vertebra. To me, scaling Everest couldn't have felt better. I gave my aching forearm a rest while Gary probed the side of the spinal canal for further bleeding. "Look, Frank"—he gently tugged the spinal cord to one side, showing a tangle of thick, oozing veins—"I think this is where the clot originated. He must have flexed his neck badly when the truck rolled over and tore one of these veins. The slow ooze gave him the progressive paralysis." He coagulated the veins with the bipolar cautery and packed the area with a small piece of Billy's back muscle.

Fred came in again at the end of the case and Gary described the findings. "Very good," said the attending surgeon, who had retreated to the far end of the room and was rummaging in an equipment drawer. Fred came over to the scrub nurses' table and opened a sterile marking pen onto the field. "What's that for?" Gary gave the staff man a quizzical stare.

"Well," observed Fred dryly, "you have such a large area of dura exposed, I thought you might want to personalize it by writing 'Fuck you, Fred,' or something like that." Both men laughed. They looked like colleagues now. I felt more like a surgeon and less like a medical student. In the glow of this male bonding, however, a question remained: How would Billy feel?

As for Walter, he wasn't feeling anything. He had been sleeping on the OR floor for the past three hours.

Billy was no better the next day, or the day after that. He was transferred to a rotating bed, designed to keep the quadriplegic patient in constant motion and prevent the formation of phlebitis and bedsores. He had regained a little motion in his biceps muscles, but his hands and legs remained paralyzed. He did retain some sensation in his stomach and feet, but not much, and he had lost bladder and bowel control.

He spent his days listening to the radio and talking with his family and friends, all the while turning about like a rack of ribs on a spit. His mood was defiant and upbeat. He talked with his son about the fishing trips they would take. His wife brought in the family finances for his approval and read the newspaper to him daily. He treated his disability as purely temporary and was determined not to let his marriage or his mind wither like his nerveless muscles.

Making rounds on patients like Billy is a difficult task. People complain about the little time their surgeons spend with them, but they should try it from our perspective. What could I say to this man—How are you feeling today? (Paralyzed from the chin down, thank you, same as yesterday.) Small talk begins to look truly small: How about that win by the Pirates? Do you think it's going to rain this weekend? Hey, time to get those tomato plants in! Eventually, however, doctor and patient find some neutral ground, some subject they can discuss that does not draw attention to the reality at hand. With Billy it was tennis.

Billy's wife told me that he was an avid tennis fan. One day in June, after Billy had been hospitalized about three weeks, I found him sitting in a stretch chair watching the French Open on TV. His neck was still wrapped in a rigid plastic collar, and his hands and feet were bound in braces to slow the formation of contractures in his lifeless limbs. He was shouting "Just keep it in, just keep it in!" at the screen.

"What are you watching?" I asked.

"Oh, Jimmy Connors playing some kid at Roland Garros. The kid is trying to play serve-and-volley against Connors on clay. Connors isn't consistent today, and if the kid would just stay back and play some longer rallies, he might do better. Right now he's getting his ass kicked. You can't play serve-and-volley on the brick dust unless you're McEnroe."

We sat and talked for an hour about pro tennis and our own philosophies about playing the game. I told him I preferred the baseline game, which surprised him. He thought my height favored a net game. He was being kind. In reality, my body habitus favors sitting in the stands with a Sno-Cone.

He grew quiet. "When do you think I'll hit a serve again?" I told him I didn't know. It was the truth: I didn't. From that day on he called me Pancho, a reference to Pancho Gonzales, the tennis great. I called him Bjorn.

Billy's huge wound eventually fell apart and became infected with pseudomonas bacteria. He developed pneumonia and an infected left kidney. Despite the rotating bed, his legs developed phlebitis. He was young and tough, however, bouncing back from each illness. One day, near the end of his acute hospitalization, something happened. Something small, but very important.

Billy had recovered from his lung problems and was in a regular hospital bed. In another day he would be transferred to the spinal cord rehabilitation unit of West Suburban Rehab Center, about five miles away. The mountains of cards he had received from friends and family had already been bundled together with twine.

"So long, Bjorn."

"Yeah, see you Pancho." He was grinning from ear to ear. "There is something I want to show you—I haven't shown anyone yet, not even my therapists."

"What's the secret?"

"Look at my left hand." I looked. I stared at it for several minutes, and then, quite subtly, almost imperceptibly, the thumb moved. "I think it's moving," Billy cried out, "it feels like it's moving. Is it moving?"

"Goddamn, Bjorn, it *is* moving! Centre Court, here you come!"

"It's not much, but maybe I'll get enough back in one hand to run a computer. If I can run a computer, maybe I can make a living again. . . ." He began to cry, I think for the first time since his truck had flipped over.

I sat down beside him. "No, Billy, if you can move a thumb, it means your spinal cord is waking up. You never had a complete injury. Who knows where this will lead. You have to work hard. When they write your story in *Reader's Digest* and use the old cliché 'Doctors said he would never walk again,' don't include me in that group, all right?"

"Fucking right." He composed himself. "Fucking right I'll work hard. Ask anybody that knows me."

I looked at his wound, still packed with cotton gauze but slowly healing. Putting a hand on his shoulder, I said goodbye and left.

Billy went to rehab, and I didn't hear anything about him for a long time. In the ensuing months, Gary went on to New York and private practice, while I left the clinical service for a one-year stint in the basic science program. One of the flaws of surgical residency is that it centers on inpatient care. We often don't get to see the small miracles that occur beyond our hospital walls.

In early January I was in neuropathology, imprisoned six days a week in my cubicle surrounded by glass slides, books, and printed handouts from our instructors. Life in pathology was dull, and I could feel blood coagulating in my veins as I sat for hour after mind-numbing hour staring at Carpenters' *Neuroanatomy* text. The pathology viewing room was empty, the attending pathologists were at the V.A. for a staff meeting, and the pathology residents, like mice when the cats are away, had bolted for the local ski slopes. I was half asleep when a tennis ball came bounding into my lap.

I looked up and saw a tall, gaunt man standing in the doorway. He looked into my puzzled face. "What's the matter, Pancho, don't you recognize me in the vertical position?"

"Jesus Christ, Billy is that you?" He was right, I didn't recognize him. The face bloated by months of steroids was now thin; the collar and braces were gone. He turned around, unbuttoned his shirt, and dropped it off his shoulders to show the jagged wound between his shoulder blades I had inflicted eight months earlier. Like doubting Thomas, I felt compelled to put my hand upon the broad scar. "I guess you did work hard, didn't you?"

"I started improving pretty rapidly after I got out of this place," he explained. "By October I was walking on the parallel bars. I went home in December. It was the best Christmas I ever had. I'm here to see Fred, and I wanted to see you guys, too. Where's Gary?"

"He's in New York making money."

"And smoking twice as much, I'm sure. It took me an hour to find you."

"How do you feel?"

"My feet still feel funny, and I can't walk as far as I would like, but I'm getting better all the time. I return to work next month." He thought for a while, then continued. "I can never look at my wife or children in the same way. That doesn't sound right ... Let's say that when Joey asks to play ball, I'll play ball as long as he wants. I don't remember everything that happened, except that it happened so fast ... so fast. It's like that sappy Christmas movie, when an angel shows some guy how the world would be without him, and then lets him go back so that he can appreciate everything more. That's how I feel. Like somebody let me go back and I can never waste a single day again." He strode away on his stiff legs.

"Somebody let me go back." Now, who wouldn't want to do *that* for a living?

9

A Bit of Hard Cheese

All neurosurgical residencies require their trainees to spend at least three months on medical neurology services. Neurologists treat the nonsurgical diseases of the nervous system: migraines, multiple sclerosis, myasthenia gravis, muscular dystrophy, and so on. At one time, neurologists saw all neurological diseases, operative or otherwise, referring away those cases in need of the surgeon's knife after an appropriate diagnosis had been made. With the advent of the CT scanner, however, the role of the neurologist in structural diseases of the brain and spine diminished greatly. The internist or general practitioner can now order a brain scan on a patient complaining of headache and, if the scan reveals a tumor, send him or her to the surgeon directly.

The straight pipeline from primary care to the neurosurgeon has created friction between neurologists and neurosurgeons. The neurologists are irritated about being bypassed in favor of surgeons too anxious (in their humble opinions) to cut the patient, while the surgeons increasingly view the neurologists' contribution to many diseases as nothing short of vestigial. The running joke among the neurosurgical residents was that neurology was a little guessing game to play while the CT films were processed.

The truth is, neurologists still play a valuable role. Not all brain afflictions yield to surgery, and neurosurgeons have little patience for nonoperative problems. As neurosurgeons, we should not mock neurology, since neurology is where our own heritage lies. Neurologists first discovered what different functions lie where in the brain, allowing surgeons some prayer of finding a brain tumor in the decades before CT scanning. A neurologist gave us cerebral angiography. Many early neurosurgeons were neurologists first. Much as I hate to admit it, neurologists understand the brain much more profoundly than most surgeons, just as an automotive engineer understands a V-8 engine better than a mechanic.

The neurosurgeon/neurologist dichotomy in brain disease is similar to the cardiac surgeon/cardiologist dichotomy in thoracic disease, or the general surgeon/internist dichotomy in abdominal disease. My old cardiac chief, Maggie, once observed that internists and other "nonprocedure-oriented" specialties stored their knowledge like sugar in great, floppy sacks and we stored ours in tiny sugar cubes. They had much more of it, but ours was more user-friendly.

In our own health center, unfortunately, the tension between the neurology and neurosurgery services was so great that our department would not permit us to do our required neurology elective with the university neurologists. In fact, they went one arrogant step further and mandated that the only neurology service good enough for *their* residents was at a London hospital. London was the birthplace of both neurology and neurosurgery. The first full-time brain surgeon in history, the great Sir Victor Horsley, practiced there.

I had no burning desire to be in London for three

months. Our department of neurosurgery "graciously" paid my airfare, but reimbursed me for nothing else. London is an expensive place to live and I could not just give up my current apartment for only three months, and so I was faced with paying rent on two residences during the rotation. This would consume all of my moonlighting money. I appealed to the department to let me do my neurology at home. They refused, and off to Merrie Olde Englande I went.

I spent my first night in London lying awake listening to the trains rumble past my bedroom window. I had an uneasy feeling, thousands of miles from home, in a country where I had no friends and no family—no one who would know if I disappeared off the face of the earth. But my discomfort soon passed. Years earlier I would have stayed terrified for weeks, but I was changing. The years of residency had begun to permeate my personality; I now looked at myself as a neurosurgeon. The James Bond feeling that sustained me in moments of clinical crisis was starting to carry over into my out-of-hospital persona as well. Endless days and nights spent summoning the nerve to stick a tube into someone's nose, a needle into someone's back, a drill into someone's skull, or a knife into someone's brain were now making it easier for me to face challenges outside the hospital as well. The next morning I confidently walked to Kensington High Street station and boarded the Circle line, headed for my first day in the birthplace of neurosurgery.

After some meandering, I finally located the quaint collection of buildings making up the London medical complex that was my final destination. The main hospital had the musty smell and vaulted ceilings of a structure dating from the previous century, with tall, wooden-framed windows still filled with original glass panes rippled by age. The walls were topped with elaborate plaster moldings. A circular stairway of trodden marble and hardwood bannisters spiraled to the first patient floor. On that floor were two large wards, male and female, each with two dozen metal-frame beds arranged in rows on either side of a long steam radiator covered by an ornate metal grill. These cavernous wards contained the neurology service.

While the foyer and hallways were heated to barely sixty degrees (considered positively balmy by U.K. standards), I found the wards to be quite warm. The increased heating of the patient-care areas was evidence that even the British didn't believe their own hogwash about lower temperatures' being "healthier." In reality, the ambient temperature was directly proportional to the robustness of the government health service's budget at the time.

This was clearly not American medicine. The wards were bigger and more chaotic than the ones at the V.A. The nurses were universally female and wore long blue and white smocks with watches pinned to the front, outfits in style during World War I. They all answered to "sister." When I first heard this title, I was confused. Was this a Catholic hospital? In the middle of Anglican London? I later learned that this was the local idiom for "nurse" and was used with respect and admiration.

One of the "sisters" introduced me to William, a tall, pasty fellow with thick wire-rimmed glasses. William was the senior neurology registrar for the ward. Registrars are the U.K. equivalent of residents, except that the position of registrar may go on indefinitely.

In the United States, residencies have a defined length. As long as a resident meets the minimum requirements for finishing, he or she is virtually guaranteed to enter the realm of attending physician at the expected time. Not so in Great Britain, where the centralized planning of socialized medicine sets the maximum number of attending jobs available. Thus, a neurology registrar can exit training only when openings for an attending neurologist become available. This occurs when an existing neurologist retires, dies, or emigrates for a larger salary—in other words, not very often.

William, at forty-five, had already held registrar positions in internal medicine, pulmonary medicine, and pediatrics. His tactic was to keep changing specialties after four or five years, as opposed to staying as a trainee in one specialty for ten to fifteen years waiting for an opening. At the present rate, he expected to retire before he finished his training. "I'm the smartest, most overtrained, and least-employed doctor in the whole bloody world," he once bitterly observed.

William's assistant registrar was David, a man of thirty. David was strikingly handsome, with a granite jaw, coal black hair, and blue eyes. He had a smooth voice and cultured accent which oozed his Oxford background.

Because it was under few financial pressures to behave otherwise, the neurology service operated at a glacial pace. The lone CT scanner was usually backed up for days, even weeks, and more involved studies were even harder to come by. The rate of patient progress was so slow that the attendings rounded only once a week, compared to once or twice a day in the United States. I would come in every morning expecting the frenetic activity I had come to associate with American inpatient care, only to find the nurses and the patients staring at one another. Watching a case unfold was like watching grass grow.

One Sunday, a middle-aged man was admitted after having a subarachnoid hemorrhage during sexual intercourse with his wife. He was in excellent condition: awake, alert, and with only a trace of headache. Back in the States, we would have performed angiography and surgery to clip the aneurysm within twenty-four hours of his arrival. But this was London. We simply tucked the man into his ward bed and scheduled his cerebral angiogram—the next slot was fourteen days away. He would have to wait. Dr. Newley, the attending neurologist, saw the patient three days after he was admitted.

"Shouldn't we get the surgeons involved?" I queried him, somewhat brashly.

He looked at me with the serene compassion of a master looking at his impudent dog. "My dear boy," he replied, "let's get the angiogram first and see what the chap's got first. I hate to bother Mr. Davies with this until we're sure." British surgeons carry the title "mister," a throwback to the days when surgeons weren't physicians but barbers, farmers, blacksmiths, or anybody else a physician could con into wielding a scalpel without benefit of anesthesia or sterile technique.

Wait and see what the "chap" has got? This calm approach to subarachnoid hemorrhage disturbed me. I was accustomed to a more aggressive management style.

The "chap" waited uneventfully through the first week. The following Sunday, though, while glancing over the sports page and eating lunch, he shouted, grabbed his head, and fell forward into his bowl of vegetable soup. He burbled into the bowl for untold minutes until one of the sisters found him. She pulled him out and started CPR, but he quickly died.

"He might have had a seizure and drowned in his soup," said William.

"Bullshit," I interjected.

"Oh, you Americans are so wonderfully blunt," William continued, "but I doubt we'll ever know what really happened."

No autopsy was performed. The following Wednesday we had weekly rounds with Dr. Newley. Afterward, the attending neurologist grabbed his overcoat and was about to leave when he suddenly turned to William and inquired about "that poor bleed fellow in the next-to-the-last bed on the right."

"Oh, yes . . . he died three days ago. Fell plop, right into his soup. Probable rebleed." William was positively blasé. I shuddered to think what the boss would say if one of his hospitalized patients had died and I had waited three days to tell him about it.

The aging neurologist passed a hand through his still-red hair and grinned wickedly. "A bit of hard cheese, those aneurysms!" He walked away and never mentioned the case again.

This was going to be a long winter.

To their credit, the neurologists, neurosurgeons, and registrars I encountered tried very hard to render good care in the face of bureaucracy, overcrowding, and chronic lack of funds and equipment. Those tasks that required little or no money to do, like taking a patient history or performing a physical examination, they did superbly and with deep attention to detail. The deficiencies in technology had sharpened their personal diagnostic acumen.

On my first day, William took me to a patient's bedside to observe the complete neurological examination on a woman with multiple sclerosis. He brought with him a large wooden box. Opening the box, he produced a small tray full of sealed vials and set it upon the patient's nightstand. As he readied his other equipment, I picked up the vials and glanced at them. They were full of liquids and powders; one was labeled "coffee," another "cloves," and yet another "vanilla."

"What are these for, William? Are we going to do some baking?"

"No," he laughed, "these are to test the young lady's sense of smell."

"Sense of smell?"

"Yes, watch." He uncapped a vial, occluded the woman's right nostril, and told her to close her eyes while inhaling with her left nostril. As she obeyed, he thrust the open vial under her nose.

"I think . . . it's orange, yes, like orange peel," said the woman without opening her eyes.

"Excellent!" said William. "See? The sense of smell is diminished in frontal-lobe tumors, particularly meningiomas of the olfactory groove. Testing for smell is often overlooked."

That was an understatement. Back at home, we *never* tested the sense of smell. But then, at home I could obtain a CT scan for an olfactory-groove tumor in less than two hours. In London, patients often waited months for elective CT scans.

As if he were performing surgery, William methodically conducted the exam over the next hour, pulling tool

after tool from his wooden box. There were test tubes
filled with hot and cold water to test temperature sensation; a compass to test two-point discrimination on various skin surfaces; a long strip of black velvet with white
stripes painted on it to test for optokinetic nystagmus; a
rotating wheel device, which looked like a pizza cutter,
to demarcate areas of decreased touch sensation; a
goniometer to measure joint flexibility; little wands with
red tips to test peripheral vision; an index card of nursery
rhymes and riddles to test mentation. Even his reflex
hammer was unique—a huge rubber wheel fixed to the
end of a two-foot-long plastic stick. It looked more like a
police weapon, or a truck tire fixed to a telephone pole,
than a medical instrument. These hammers were standard
issue in London. William claimed that the only way to
test reflexes was to hit the limbs with "real momentum."

The history-taking on the neurology service was
equally fastidious. One afternoon, after taking a history
from a man with headaches, I was grilled by the hospital's chief neurologist on teaching rounds.

"What does Mr. Hughes do for a living, Doctor?" the
kindly professor asked.

"He says he works in a shop," I replied. At home, that
would have been the end of the discussion on that topic.

"What sort of shop?"

"I don't know, some sort of small store, maybe."

"Well, what sort of shop might make a difference,
don't you think? If he works in a paint store all day
mixing paint with hydrocarbon thinners, might not that
be a cause of his headaches?"

"Well, yes," I admitted.

"Does he own the shop?"

"I don't know."

The professor removed his glasses and began cleaning them slowly, squinting up at the high ceiling as he continued his dissertation. "These facts matter a great deal. What a patient does for a living, what his background is, what level of education he has achieved . . . all of these issues must be addressed in great detail in order to put his complaints and his disease in the proper context. If I ask a man to take the square root of 100 and he cannot, I might take this as proof of a left-hemispheric brain tumor, unless I know that he has worked on a farm since childhood and never attended school. Likewise, I might find it normal that a patient could not tell me the current exchange rate of the pound in Japanese yen. But if I knew that person was a merchant banker, on the other hand, ignorance of this fact would indicate a grave illness indeed! Americans have grown so dependent upon their scanning toys that they fail to view the patient as a multi-dimensional person. To have the audacity to cut into a person's brain without the slightest clue of his life, his occupation . . . I find that most simply appalling."

These words came back to me years later in the States. I was operating on a woman for a spinal tumor when a medical student in the room casually asked me how old the patient was. I couldn't remember! Here I was, staring at the woman's spinal cord, and I didn't even know how old she was! The professor was right; it was most simply appalling. I was treating an MRI image on a piece of photographic film, not a person. I've tried hard not to repeat that arrogance again.

Multiple sclerosis, or MS, is more common in the U.K. than it is in the United States, and we saw a great deal of it during my three months in London. The disease affects the insulating fat, or myelin, around nerve fibers, punching holes (called plaques) into the deep white matter of the brain and spinal cord. The severity of the disease depends upon where the plaques occur. A large plaque in a tolerant area of the brain, such as the right frontal lobe, may be asymptomatic, while a minuscule plaque in a critical area of the spinal cord or brain stem may leave the patient wheelchair-bound.

MS is capricious, striking quickly and then retreating in a series of random exacerbations scattered over a lifetime. The patient may be disabled for months, then recover and be unaffected for years before another episode occurs. At the time I was doing my neurology rotation, there was no accepted treatment save for high-dose steroids and physical therapy. (Other therapies are now available, such as interferon.) For most patients, fortunately, the tincture of time was the best cure.

The most dramatic MS patient I ever saw was Andrew, a Nigerian foreign exchange student at the University of London. He was admitted with his very first attack of the illness. The hospital's newly installed MRI scanner (dedicated by the Prince of Wales himself!) disclosed a half-inch plaque dead-center in his midbrain. The midbrain sits atop the brain stem, where it serves as a conduit for the output of the hindbrain cerebellum, the main balance and coordination computer of the brain. This output had been effectively amputated by the plaque, leaving Andrew with no cerebellar function at all.

The cerebellum, or "little cerebrum," fine-tunes the gross motor signals emanating from the upper brain. Its output is purely inhibitory: the neurons in the cerebellum serve only to dampen or inhibit the activity of other neurons in the brain. My neuroanatomy professor in medical school put this into perspective by observing that Michelangelo had carved the statue of David using only "subtraction" of stone. Thus, the big cerebrum's motor outflow is like raw marble which the cerebellum deftly chisels into coordinated movements.

As long as Andrew kept very still, he was fine. However, the moment he tried to do even the slightest task, even to scratch his nose, his arms and legs became uncontrollable, flailing about like octopus tentacles. He had to be fed, since he could not be trusted with a fork or knife. His face was swollen from attempts to brush his teeth, attempts which resulted only in a self-inflicted pummeling. He could walk short distances, but his gait was wild. More often than not, he ended up draped over the ward's central radiator, crying from frustration.

This uncoordinated movement, called ataxia, even involved Andrew's speech. Although the melodic Nigerian inflections of his perfect English were still detectable, the words came out herky-jerky, with the tone monotonous and the sentences incorrectly parsed, a pattern known as cerebellar scanning speech. Scanning speech has a hollow, mechanical quality, like the diction of robots and computers in science fiction films. Like the stare of the acute schizophrenic, scanning speech is difficult to describe in words, but once you have experienced it you remember it forever.

As we sat drinking our afternoon coffee (we still called it "tea time," although few registrars actually drank tea), William, David, and I watched Andrew as he ricocheted around the ward, walking into beds and walls and bouncing away in a different direction like a mechanical toy.

"Poor bastard," remarked David.

"Not to worry," observed William, "he'll get better.

They all do from the first episode, no matter how bloody awful they look. In six or eight months he'll be back at school again. The question is how to manage him until this plaque remits. The physical therapy people have fitted him for a lead jacket."

"A lead jacket?" I asked.

William continued. "Yes, a lead jacket. It's a suit coat that's been fitted with lead bars to make the arms very heavy. If Andrew has to work harder to move his arms and gets more proprioceptive feedback from them, he can control his movements a little better. Quit beating himself up all of the time. It's quite low-tech, you know, but it works."

"The main drawback," added David, "is they get dreadfully tired, as you can well imagine. Ah, but just think! If he wears it for a few months, he may end up looking like the Incredible Hulk!"

The jacket was delivered the following day. It was of heavy green cloth and looked identical to the protective "burner's jackets" worn by the acetylene torch operators in the steel mill. Numerous slots were sewn along the arms. Along with the jacket came a carton of thin lead bars to be placed into the slots, allowing us to titrate the added weight so that we could give Andrew some motor control without rendering him unable to lift his arms at all.

We spent the morning experimenting with the jacket, until finally Andrew was able to lift his arm, slowly and agonizingly, and run a comb through his short hair. His mouth blossomed into a broad African grin.

"Ah, this is very much more to my liking!" he said in his robot voice, beaming at his regained arm control.

He could only wear the jacket a few hours at a time,

and by the end of each day his arms ached so much that he had to take narcotics to sleep. But he stopped crying the day he got the jacket. As William predicted, Andrew's speech slowly returned to normal, his drunken gait began to sober, and his need for the jacket diminished weekly. Two months after he came to us a limp jellyfish of a man, the Nigerian strode out the hospital door, erect and controlled, the only remnant of his disease the increased power in his well-exercised arms. He shook our hands briskly.

"You know, I am a philosophy student," Andrew observed just as he exited, flexing his biceps in a body-builder's pose. "Nietzsche said 'Whatever doesn't kill me makes me stronger.' I now know this as fact. Thank you, my friends."

He would be back, no doubt—in a year, maybe ten, depending upon the mercy of his personal disease. Had we, as Hippocrates postulated, simply "entertained" Andrew until he got better on his own? Perhaps, but we had managed to stop his tears, and any therapy which accomplishes that feat for a suffering patient is damned good medicine.

The U.K. is hardly a classless society. Nevertheless, I was amazed at the degree to which nationality, race, and socioeconomic status factored into and at times hindered the clinical reasoning of the registrars and attending neurologists.

London has a very large number of people from the Indian subcontinent, a vestige of the days of the empire. Whenever recent immigrants from India or Pakistan showed up at our doorstep, they were immediately given the diagnosis of tuberculosis, regardless of their symptoms. A middle-aged Pakistani grocer, for example, came to the casualty department (British for ER) with a three-month history of progressive weakness and stiffness in his legs. An MRI scan revealed a mass within the center of his thoracic spinal cord, between the shoulder blades. I recognized it as an astrocytoma, a tumor arising from the spinal tissues. To my chagrin, the attending surgeon, Mr. Royston, diagnosed it as a tuberculoma, a swelling caused by the tuberculosis bacterium, even though the patient had a negative chest X ray and no other evidence or history of tuberculosis. The patient's nationality was cited as the sole reason for this bizarre conclusion.

I went to the library the next day and could unearth only two previous cases of a solitary tuberculous mass in the spinal cord, and both of those reported cases had documented pulmonary TB. When I confronted the surgeon with this fact, he shrugged and pointed to the good clinical response the patient had made to the antituberculous antibiotics as further proof of the correctness of the original diagnosis. The patient truly *was* better, but I argued that the improvement could be from the steroid medication that was being administered as well. I made no headway. Three weeks later, the patient returned to the casualty department in a state of near-paraplegia and emergency surgery was performed, at which time his astrocytoma was removed and he made an uneventful recovery.

In another incident, we were gathered to hear a patient demonstration by one of the most senior and respected neurologists in all of southern England. Donning our white jackets, I and the other trainees crammed into the archaic demonstration hall, sitting in ascending concentric circles around the small exam table below. A registrar brought in the patient, a scrawny laborer in his fifth decade. The patient staggered to the table and sat down, but proceeded to bob and sway even while seated. The stately neurologist conducted a detailed interview with the man, listening keenly to his complaints: unsteady gait, dizziness, and nausea. He conducted a very cursory exam and then had the patient escorted from the lecture hall. The neurologist turned to us, paused for a dramatic effect, and asked, "What single piece of information you have heard this morning tells you what is wrong with this man?"

"His age," answered a registrar.

"No, that's not correct."

"His occupation?" I volunteered.

"No, wrong once again."

This continued for a few minutes, until the exasperated teacher told us his expected answer: "His nationality! His name is O'Brien and he's from Belfast. Since he's obviously of the Irish lower classes, it's a very good bet that he's a sot. He's clearly afflicted with alcoholic cerebellar degeneration."

In fact, this diagnosis was correct, but the bluntness of this deduction would not have been tolerated in America. The neurologist never even asked the patient if he drank; he simply assumed it to be true. I couldn't see one of our neurologists standing before an open forum of medical students and announcing that a patient must be a user of crack cocaine simply because he was black and from an urban area.

"I can't see!" The woman spoke in a measured tone, trying to conceal her panic in proper British fashion.

"Keep calm and tell us what's been going on," William reassured her.

The patient, a pretty young woman still wearing her street clothes, arrived on the neurology ward just as we were returning from lunch at a local pub. The casualty department, where she had gone seeking help for progressive blindness, had sent her directly to our service.

"I was fine this morning when I woke up, but after breakfast I began having a headache, right here." She motioned to the top of her head. "My vision began to blur, but I could still see well enough to get here. Now I can only see dark forms moving about, and things are getting darker all the time!"

William turned to David and me, speaking in low tones. "David, notify the CT scan facility that we will need an immediate pituitary study. Frank, go to the Jefferson ward and find Mr. Cunningham and bring him here at once. Quickly now." Mr. Cunningham was a senior attending surgeon and the hospital's pituitary specialist.

I dashed off to the Jefferson ward and found Mr. Cunningham in his office; we were back on the neurology ward within minutes. The young woman, Alice Weathers, recounted her story to the surgeon. Her health was good, although her menstrual periods had become irregular during the preceding year and she had noticed a slight discharge from her nipples recently. Unmarried, she typed for a living and lived alone in the Tottenham Court area.

Mr. Cunningham examined her vision. She could make out his large hand waving in front of her face, but she could not count his fingers or tell the color of his necktie. The surgeon's elegant face turned dour.

"Young lady," he began, "I believe that a tumor has hemorrhaged within your pituitary gland, that small bit of tissue located behind your eyes. We call this hemor-rhaging 'pituitary apoplexy.' The blood clot is pushing on the optic nerves, the nerves that connect the eyes to the brain. I will have to operate immediately to remove the clot and tumor or you will remain blind."

"Tumor? I have cancer?"

"No, no, my dear young lady. The tumor is almost cer-tainly a benign adenoma, a growth quite common in young women. In your case, the tumor is making a hormone called prolactin. Excess prolactin hormone will produce exactly the symptoms you have noted—the irregular menstruation, the slight nipple discharge. That discharge is milk. Prolactin is a hormone normally made during pregnancy. It stimulates the fatty breast tissue to manu-facture milk."

"Do what you have to do, just don't let me go blind. Please!"

Mr. Cunningham examined the patient's breasts and confirmed the milk secretion. "Have her taken to the operating theaters straightaway and cancel the scan. There is little doubt what needs to be done here. I will scan her after I have decompressed the optic nerves. Be sure to administer a large dose of hydrocortisone, won't you? I will have my senior registrar lend a hand."

I followed the patient to the holding area outside the operating suite. She wept quietly into a handful of tissues.

"Is there anyone I can call to be with you?" I asked.

"My dad died two years ago and my mum's got a bad heart. I'd rather not tell her anything right now."

I couldn't begin to imagine her despair as she faced this crisis alone. After several minutes of waiting, an OR nurse whisked her into the room and an anesthesiologist ended her suffering with a whiff of gas.

Little more than fifty minutes had passed since she had arrived in the casualty department. British medicine at its finest. Although mired in red tape, the U.K. system avoids the legal wrangling that hamstrings American medicine. In the United States, taking a woman to the OR without objective studies, such as MRI or CT scans, invites malpractice action should anything go wrong. True, Gary had cut Billy's spine without a myelogram, but such fortitude is rare. Back home, anesthesia would balk at doing her so soon after she had eaten breakfast. And the operating rooms would have been overbooked. In London, the mighty Mr. Cunningham spoke and things happened.

Mr. Cunningham and his registrar positioned Alice in the head clamp, then scrubbed her mouth and nose with soap. The pituitary, an embryonic relic of the nasal passages, lies buried in the hard palate, just above the uvula. The neurosurgeon approaches the gland through the nose, with the aid of a microscope and some truly long instruments. To enter the hypophysis (the correct name for the gland), the surgeon traverses the sphenoid sinus; hence the operation's tongue-twisting name—transsphenoidal hypophysectomy.

First used by Cushing in the early twentieth century, the transsphenoidal procedure is arguably the most bizarre operation in the neurosurgeon's repertoire. To enter the nose, the surgeon cuts under the upper lip and peels the face up and away from the "nares," the openings of the nasal passages. Cracking the nasal septum to one side, the surgeon advances a large speculum to the base of the skull, the sphenoid sinus is removed, and the floor of the pituitary chamber is chiseled away.

Cushing had little luck with this approach and abandoned it, preferring to take the tumors out through the head rather than down through the nose. Superb a technician though he was, Cushing lacked a microscope, and the fiber-optic lighting, needed to do the operation safely. Jules Hardy and his colleagues in Canada resurrected the procedure in the 1960s, with superb results, and the nasal approach soon became standard. Hardy's use of the microscope and intraoperative X rays overcame Cushing's difficulties.

Mr. Cunningham deftly dissected the pretty woman's face and exposed her pituitary gland in less than an hour. The gland looked blue and taut on the video screen. With a swift poke of his pointed microblade, thick clot and purulent yellow tumor gushed from the gland and into Mr. Cunningham's thin suction tip. He spent several minutes rummaging around with small currettes, until satisfied that all tumor and blood clot were evacuated. The task of reassembling the face fell to the registrar.

Alice's broad smile in the recovery room told more about her eyes than any formal vision test could do. A few hours after surgery, her vision returned to normal. The nasal packing was removed on the third postoperative day and she went home on the fifth—pretty as ever. Her mother never learned of Alice's brief flirtation with disaster.

The day of her apoplexy, as I was fetching Mr. Cunningham from his office, I noticed a wooden plaque on the surgeon's wall. It read prophetically: SOMETIMES SURGERY DOES HELP.

I returned to the United States shortly after Alice went home. My first assignment was Children's Hospital, where surgery often did not help at all.

10

Rebecca

On my return from England, the department assigned me to the division of pediatric neurosurgery at the local children's hospital. The pediatric rotation was unpopular among the neurosurgery residents. Drawing blood from a wailing infant in the middle of the night while the mother screams "You're murdering my baby" was just one reason. The place did have one selling point: it *wasn't* the pain service.

The neurosurgical floor in Children's Hospital was more of a Sesame Street advertisement than a clinical ward. Bert and Ernie stared down from every wall like Muppet versions of Big Brother. In the middle of the ward was the treatment room, where minor procedures were performed. The very name of that place suggested an interrogation chamber. Muppet stuffed animals littered the place, as if they could soothe a child lying strapped to a table awaiting the cold steel of a needle. Once, as I was having a particularly difficult time getting blood from an infant, I kept smacking my head against a Muppet mobile which was dangling from the light fixture. Driven nearly mad by the infant's screaming, I pulled the contraption from the light, heaved it into the corner of the room, and shouted "Fuck you, Cookie Monster!"

The infamous "swinging chairs," in which infants rocked for hours on end, lined the halls. Nurses had the audacity to call me when one of the pendular infants puked. "Let me put you in a swinging chair for a couple of hours," I would sneer, "and see how much of your lunchtime hoagie *you* keep down."

A child's cry pierces to the bone and aggravates the soul far out of proportion to its decibel level. The crying of a sick child is far worse. Eric put crying into perspective for me: "When you go to draw blood on a two-month-old, remember, he doesn't know it's just a simple procedure. He thinks you're trying to *kill* him! He's going to peg the meter, pull out all the organ stops."

Three weeks into my tour of pediatric duty, I met Rebecca, the only child of a rural couple from out of state. A free clinic had transferred the six-week-old infant to our emergency room that morning for evaluation of her lethargy, vomiting, and failure to gain weight. A CT scan, ordered by the ER pediatrician, revealed a tumor in Rebecca's small brain. As the neurosurgical resident on call, I was summoned to admit her for further treatment.

I found Rebecca with her parents in the ER's cast room, a cluttered cubicle used for setting bones and placing plaster casts. The cast room also doubled as a holding area for ER patients awaiting hospital admission. The infant, wearing only a plastic diaper and soiled T-shirt, squirmed in her mother's lap and gummed a pink pacifier.

Both parents sported worn denim clothes and looked to be no older than twenty. Father paced the small room puffing a cigarette, while mother stared quietly at the floor, her pale face framed by straight, bleached hair.

Rebecca's appearance startled me. Her bulbous, over-sized head teetered unsteadily atop a tiny body, the scalp stretched to a porcelain sheen and laced with delicate blue veins. An intravenous line, anchored by a piece of yellow Big Bird tape, dangled from a scalp vein. Her rib cage bulged beneath the parchment skin of her chest. Her eyes deviated so far downward that only small crescents of her watery-blue irises were visible. The exposed white of her eyes, together with the gaunt, corrugated chest and large head, endowed Rebecca with a pitiful, buglike aspect—typical of untreated infantile hydrocephalus.

Hydrocephalus, Greek for "water brain," results from a blockage of normal cerebrospinal-fluid flow within the brain. CSF moistens and cushions the gelatinous nervous tissue. One pint of CSF is made in the brain daily, percolating through small chambers and tunnels within the head and spine before flowing back to the brain's surface, where it is absorbed by large veins.

CSF production is relentless, a faucet with no "off" position. Any obstacle to CSF flow causes fluid accumulation, increasing the pressure on the brain. A variety of diseases causes hydrocephalus. The viscous pus of meningitis, for example, plugs the tiny CSF channels like grease clogging a kitchen trap. Intrauterine infections, including cytomegalovirus and toxoplasmosis, scar the fetal brain's inner cavities and produce a form of congenital hydrocephalus.

Rebecca's hydrocephalus stemmed from a blockage of the fourth ventricle, the main drainage pathway within the brain. A tumor in her cerebellum, the crinkled hindbrain, was the culprit.

Because the mature skull is solid bone, adult-onset hydrocephalus slowly crushes the brain between pressurized fluid and the skull. The infant skull, on the other hand, is pliable, consisting of eggshell-thin plates of bone linked by fibrous fontanelles, or "soft spots." Designed to expand slowly during normal brain growth, the baby's skull offers little resistance to unchecked accumulation of CSF. If untreated, infantile hydrocephalus inflates a head to freakish proportions, transforming the brain into a translucent water balloon.

While hydrocephalus remains common in children, modern treatments using surgically implanted plastic shunts have reduced monstrous heads to textbook oddities, although in some rural areas, where access to medical care is limited, advanced cases of untreated hydrocephalus still exist. About once a year, a child with a grotesque head is trundled into our medical center, carried on a wagon or cart like a human watermelon. Children with uncontrolled hydrocephalus look more like Hollywood-created space aliens than human beings, with massive foreheads bulging out over tiny faces.

Hydrocephalus damages brain mechanisms controlling eye movements, deviating the eyes downward. The exaggerated downward gaze is called "sunsetting," since only the top portions of the irises are visible. The brain's nausea center, when compressed by hydrocephalus, signals frequent, forceful vomiting, with subsequent dehydration of the patient. In Rebecca's case, her inability to hold down food spurred her parents to seek medical attention.

Rebecca was not irreversibly deformed, not yet anyway. But she was in serious trouble. I approached her parents, the Hobsons, with my best professional demeanor.

"I'm Dr. Vertosick, Mr. and Mrs. Hobson, from neurosurgery," I said as I strode into the room, Rebecca's

X-ray jacket under my arm. This introduction garnered only quizzical stares.

"Neurosurgery?" asked Mr. Hobson.

"We're the brain surgeons," I continued, hoping to clarify the obviously unfamiliar term "neurosurgeon." I disliked the label "brain surgeon." It evoked silly images of Jethro Bodine, bearer of a sixth-grade education.

"Brain surgeon! What do we need a brain surgeon for?" cried the mother. She held Rebecca closer, as if to keep her out of my clutches. This family had no clue—no one had bothered to tell them about the scan.

"Your daughter—Rebecca, is it?—her scan shows a growth, a growth in her brain. That's why she's been spitting up all the time." "Growth" is a good word, much better than "tumor," or "cancer."

Dad ground out his cigarette under the heel of a weathered boot. "What sort of growth?"

"A lump, growing in the back of the brain—here," I explained, touching the velvety nape of Rebecca's tiny neck, "about the size of a grape."

Foods are the traditional yardstick for tumors anywhere in the body. "A tumor the size of" a grape, walnut, egg, melon, orange. Although a macabre practice, food comparisons allow a visceral feel for prognosis—someone with a cancerous cantaloupe in their chest isn't going to live as long as someone with a cancerous pea. Although a "grape-sized" brain tumor doesn't seem threatening, it's plenty big enough to kill an infant.

"It may be benign," I went on, "something we could successfully remove, or it might be something that we ... uh, we can't remove completely." I can't bring myself to use the word "malignant." At least not during the initial confrontation with patients or their parents.

People faint from hearing such words. My calm assurances were deceitful. I knew that infants almost never have benign brain tumors.

I coaxed Mrs. Hobson into telling me her baby's brief history. Born after an uneventful pregnancy, Rebecca was fine for about a week before her vomiting began. A clinic pediatrician in their home state advised changing formulas, thinking the child was developing a food intolerance. This strategy worked for one or two days, but the vomiting soon resumed.

After one month of life, Rebecca weighed less than she did at birth. Her head grew large as her body withered. Since Rebecca's father was unemployed and without health care coverage, they avoided further medical care and tried to correct the problem themselves, feeding the infant herbal teas, whiskey and water, orange drink, ginger ale—anything they thought she might hold down. Nothing worked. When Rebecca grew stuporous from dehydration, the parents finally agreed to come to us for help.

After examining the baby, I mumbled some additional words of encouragement to her shaking parents and left the room to call Dr. Wilson, the attending neurosurgeon on the case.

"It's a cerebellar mass, lateral, enhancing, about two centimeters," I told Dr. Wilson over the phone, holding the scan films over my head to illuminate them with the ceiling lights. "Big-time hydrocephalus, huge vents, sunsetting, the works. She'll need to be done soon."

"Yeah, sounds like it," he replied. I could hear him shuffling through some papers. "I have to give a deposition tomorrow, so put her on for Wednesday. We may need the microscope, maybe not . . . and schedule some brain-stem evoked potentials. How old is she? . . . Six weeks? Not good, not good. Must be a PNET." PNET stood for primitive neuroectodermal tumor, a tumor of the embryonic tissue which gives rise to the neurons, or nerve cells, of the brain.

I returned to the cast room. Rebecca was crying: not the penetrating wail of a healthy baby, but the weak, cat-like meowing of a brain-impaired newborn. Her mother's eyes were puffy and red as well. Her quaking fingers fumbled to replace Rebecca's now discarded binky. She must have spent most of the last six weeks trying to settle her starving baby in this way, and the strain of her sleep-lessness was palpable.

"I'll take you up to the neuro floor. Dr. Wilson will be your staff surgeon and he'll talk with you later. We don't plan to do anything more today, other than give her IV fluids and some steroid medication to make her feel better."

I glanced at my watch: lunchtime. There wasn't much more I could, or would, tell them at that time. I left them there, alone. Two adolescent parents and their dying child.

The goals of Rebecca's surgery were to relieve her hydrocephalus by removing the obstructing tumor and to confirm the diagnosis of brain cancer. If the hydro-cephalus persisted after tumor removal, a permanent shunt would be necessary. The shunt consisted of a thin plastic tube, inserted just beneath the skin, to redirect excess CSF to the abdominal cavity.

Surgery on an infant brain can be a nightmarish affair. While the adult brain is soft as warm gelatin, the infant brain is even softer. What little rigidity the brain has derives from the tough insulating fat known as myelin. Myelin first appears during the third or fourth month of life, and continues forming until the nervous system reaches full maturity at age twenty-five. A neuroanatomy professor once lamented to me that twenty-one was too young an age to vote, given that the brain wasn't even "done" yet.

At six weeks of age, the unmyelinated brain is thick soup which can be inadvertently vacuumed away by operative suctions. Moreover, nerves the thickness of pencil lead in adults are little more than a spider's web in a baby.

Infant surgery poses other problems. The loss of a thimbleful of blood, not enough to make a decent stain on a gauze sponge, sends an infant into shock. Worse still, infants are prone to fatal hypothermia. The operating room must be kept very warm. Even the IV fluids must be at the proper temperature to avoid cooling the infant excessively. The exquisite difficulties of infant surgery have a Darwinian explanation: nature doesn't want sick babies to have surgery, but to be buried. Civilization no longer cares about survival of the fittest, however. We want all our babies to live.

Dr. Wilson and I took Rebecca to the operating room on Wednesday, as planned. After she was anesthetized and a breathing tube was inserted into her throat, she was wrapped in foil to retain her body heat. These foil wraps gave us our affectionate nickname for sick infants: hoagies.

Since her tumor was in the rear position of her brain, we flipped Rebecca into the prone position, with her face resting on a padded "horseshoe" head holder. In adults, we would use a pin-and-clamp head holder known as the

Mayfield device to suspend the head in midair. The horseshoe, on the other hand, is just a modified pillow. In long operations, pressure from the horseshoe breaks down the skin, causing blisters, pressure sores, even permanent facial scarring. The thin infant skull cannot support the Mayfield clamp, however, making the risks of the horseshoe unavoidable.

Skin ulceration during prolonged operations is just one example of how anesthesia differs from sleep. During sleep, we change positions every hour, protecting each body area from prolonged pressure. When injured by a contorted position, a limb becomes painful and numb, forcing us to move or even awaken. During brain operations, such sudden movements could cause the surgeon to slip, with devastating results. For safety, the patient must be kept absolutely motionless for hours.

For long operations, we position patients with extreme care, filling eyes with ointment, padding nerves, covering intravenous tubes with soft foam.

After the baby was positioned to our satisfaction, I began shaving her downy hair, using a straight razor. This resident's job took as much skill as the surgery itself. Rebecca's scalp was just a few millimeters thick—a careless swipe and the blade could cut to the bone.

Dr. Wilson counted any nicks made during shaving. He charged us a quarter a nick, paid as one lump sum into the residents' research fund at the end of our rotation. Rebecca's head shave cost me a dollar, but I made no major razor blunders.

We would be working near Rebecca's brain stem, the upper part of her spinal cord. The brain stem, the brain's chief switchboard, is easily damaged. To monitor its function during surgery, we would use Rebecca's sense of hearing.

Sounds are transmitted from the hearing nerves into the brain via the brain stem. Thus, hearing can be used as a barometer of brain stem injury. Of course, infants, anesthetized or awake, cannot tell the surgeon whether they can hear, so hearing must be checked electronically.

To do this, small earphones emitting sharp clicking noises are taped to the patient's ears. Sound transmitted from the ear into the brain stem travels upward into the cerebrum, the "thinking" part of the brain. By attaching electrodes to the scalp overlying the hearing regions of the cerebrum, neurophysiologists can detect the subtle brain waves that occur when signals carrying the clicks arrive in our consciousness—even if we are asleep or anesthetized. Using an operating-room computer, the neurophysiologist calculates the time interval for the clicking noise to go from ear to cerebrum. Too long a transit time means that surgical injury has occurred to the brain stem or auditory nerves.

Our neurophysiologist for the day was Bob, a small, bearded man with a Ph.D. in electrical engineering, as well as an M.D.—and a ponytail. He looked like he'd just walked out of the 1960s. During the surgery he sat on his stool, gazing at a fluorescent computer screen filled with white waveforms. His warnings would give us time to adjust anything that might be injuring the brain stem before the injury became permanent.

We retired to the scrub sink as Bob finished sewing his electrodes into Rebecca's scalp and placing earphones into her small ears. We lathered our arms and hands in silence. I gazed through the OR window at the surgical tech as she painted Rebecca's misshapen head with the gooey orange Betadine. Only weeks into my rotation on this service and I already hated pediatric neurosurgery. Before each case, my mind conjured up laughing babies cuddled by their kindly grandfathers. Everybody's little bundles of joy. None of them belonged here.

Fifteen minutes later, Dr. Wilson sank his number 15 knife blade into Rebecca's scalp. The room filled with the high-pitched wailing of the suctions. As he opened a four-inch incision down the midline of Rebecca's head, I quickly placed plastic clips over the skin edges to halt the oozing. An electric knife stripped the neck muscles away from the underlying skull and cervical vertebrae. The muscle sizzled from the heat, flooding the room with the acrid smell of burning human flesh, an odor that has caused more than a few medical students to swoon. With the bone exposed, a steel Weitlaner clamp spread the wound open.

We drilled small holes into Rebecca's thin skull and used heavy scissors to pry open a bony window into the cerebellar region. The glistening white dura matter pulsated through the skull defect we had fashioned.

Before incising the dura and exposing the cerebellum, we drilled another small hole just slightly higher than our bone window and inserted a temporary drainage tube into the distended spinal-fluid sacs. Clear fluid spurted from the tube under pressure as I passed it into the brain. We were finally ready to expose the brain. We paused as the circulating nurse put on our loupes, custom-made eyeglasses with telescopic lenses that provide a threefold magnification of vision.

Dr. Wilson grasped the dura with a long forceps and nicked it with a pointed knife until the pinkish cerebellar surface peeked through. We enlarged the dural opening with fine-tipped scissors, stopping intermittently to place silver clips across small venous channels.

"Evoked potentials have improved," Bob said softly from behind the wires that engulfed him like technicolor linguini. By letting off CSF with the drainage tube, we had relieved some of the existing pressure on Rebecca's brain stem. This improvement was to be short-lived.

Rebecca's tumor showed itself as we peeled the dura away from the left side of her cerebellum. Firmer than the surrounding brain tissue, the mass was darker pink, almost purple in areas. The dura stuck to it, and tiny rivulets of blood began streaming from the tumor's raw surface as we stripped the dura away using a metal dissector.

"Cottonoids up, please." The scrub nurse brought up a gleaming steel basin full of white cotton squares of various sizes. To each square was attached a long green string. These cottonoid patties stopped our suctions from plunging into the soft brain, like snowshoes which keep feet from sinking into snow. The strings allowed the patties to be identified and removed before the case ended.

Dr. Wilson encircled the tumor with half-inch patties, holding the cottonoids with a forceps in his right hand while using a suction tip in his left hand to push the cotton squares between the tumor and the normal brain. He began developing the "plane" between tumor and cerebellum. In benign tumors, a clear plane exists and the tumor can often be popped out using this encircling technique.

In malignant tumors, however, the cancer invades deeply into normal tissue, obscuring the plane between tumor and brain. Such was the case here. As we tried to separate the tumor away from the brain, the purplish lump disintegrated and the bleeding increased. A small

piece of the friable mass was handed off to the circulating nurse in a small plastic cup for a "frozen section."
The pathologist would freeze the tumor and examine it
under a microscope to assess malignancy.

The patties were now soaked with blood and the
wound swam in the growing ooze. We aspirated the
tumor with our suctions in the vain hope that removing it
would slow the hemorrhage. Unfortunately, this maneuver
only created a deeper hole from which the red blood
continued to pour. I glanced at the heart monitor.
Rebecca's heart rate climbed steadily, a sign of her persistent blood loss.

The nurse-anesthetist called for the anesthesiologist to
return to the room.

"Trouble?" Dr. Wilson asked.

"Her pressure's dropping a bit."

"Do we have blood in the room?"

"No."

"Get some," he said sternly while shoving a large ball
of cotton wadding into the bleeding brain wound, "and
start warming it." The bleeding was getting ahead of us.

"Evoked potentials, two milliseconds out on the left,"
chimed Bob. The hearing impulses from the left ear were
taking longer to reach the upper brain regions, the first
warning of brain injury.

The surgeon shook his head. "Shit."

Although the large packing slowed the bleeding, the
pressure on the brain stem was unacceptable. If we took
out the packing Rebecca might bleed to death; leave it in
and the brain stem might be damaged, causing permanent
deafness or paralysis.

"Fuck the evoked potentials. I'm leaving this pack in

for a while, until they get some blood into her," Dr. Wilson whispered to me. Several minutes went by.

"Where's my blood?" Dr. Wilson grew restless.

"Potentials out four milliseconds on the left and the waveform is flattening," intoned Bob, a voice of doom in the corner, "and the right is now out one millisecond." The brain stem cried to Bob's computers, pleading for relief. Dr. Wilson sighed and pulled the cotton wadding from the hole. The bleeding resumed, but more slowly. I grasped the bipolar coagulator, a long forceps hooked to a battery pack which is used to coagulate small blood vessels with heat, and attacked those bleeding arteries I could identify in the soupy tumor bed.

The OR door swung open and a small, squat man dressed in white paper coveralls entered the room. The pathologist.

Dr. Wilson greeted him. "What do you have for me?"

"It's pleomorphic, highly cellular, aggressive . . . a PNET, most likely."

"Yeah, that's what we thought."

"Looks like you're up to your ass in alligators!" The pathologist's grin shone clearly from beneath his surgical mask as he glanced at the tangled mass of cottonoid strings spewing from the bloody cranial wound.

"It's a wet son of a bitch, all right," replied Dr. Wilson as he turned back to the wound, "but we'll manage."

"I'm sure you will, John," the pathologist said over his shoulder as he headed for the door, "but cases like these remind me of why I only deal with dead people."

We fell into a silent routine, sucking away bits of the tumor, stopping the bleeding, then removing more tumor. The gutted cerebellum collapsed upon itself. I held it away with thin copper "brain ribbons" as Dr. Wilson chased the tumor further and further into the depths of Rebecca's head. Downward into disaster.

Rebecca had a cancerous brain tumor. The standard methods of dealing with cancer, radiation and chemotherapy, cannot be used in infants. Radiation therapy would destroy the developing brain cells and guarantee that Rebecca would be vegetative before she reached one year of age. The single weapon we could fire at this tumor was our surgery. Removing as much tumor as we could was her only, albeit slim and very risky, chance of meaningful survival. Rebecca became hypotensive and hypothermic, her heart flipped in and out of ventricular tachycardia (one step removed from full cardiac arrest), and yet we pressed on.

"Oh, damn!" Dr. Wilson finally exclaimed as he halted the tumor resection. I peered into the hole left vacant by the excised tumor. At the bottom, spinal fluid welled up and diaphonous strands of severed nerves floated in the watery pool like minuscule bits of white seaweed. He had gone completely through the cerebellum and into the space surrounding the brain stem, where vital cranial nerves exit on their way to the ears, face, and throat. Some of the nerves were destroyed, meaning that Rebecca might not hear, swallow, or breathe after surgery. The aggressive tumor resection was a gamble which we had lost.

"The left evoked potentials are out completely," Bob said, his computers verifying the damage we could see with our eyes. The hearing nerve was transected on the left side.

Dr. Wilson put a cotton ball into the tumor bed and squinted at the CT scan hanging on a view box across the room, trying to compose himself. He was motionless for a long time. I have since come to know the agony of those minutes which follow hurting someone badly in the operating room. In those moments, the fear of confronting the family, the panicked thoughts of changing careers, visions of lawyers—all dance through the mind in a flash.

"Surgicel." He finally stirred and called for the fine cellulose mesh used to fill the tumor bed. Done. Tumor remained in the cerebellum, but Wilson had lost his stomach for this case. With an incompletely resected PNET and several damaged cranial nerves, Rebecca was officially unsalvageable. Outside the OR, in a smoke-filled room, Rebecca's parents and grandparents waited for good news that would never come. There would be no prom for Rebecca. We packed the brain with wads of surgicel and sutured the dura closed without speaking another word.

We took Rebecca to the recovery room still asleep and on a ventilator. She made a few decerebrate movements with her arms and confirmed our worst fear: we had damaged the stem. Decerebration, a rigid posture of the limbs, indicates a living, but dysfunctional, brain stem.

We called the family into a more private conference room, away from the crowded OR waiting area. I sat in a corner of the room as Dr. Wilson explained the situation to Rebecca's parents and maternal grandparents. Unlike television, where people take bad news with explosive histrionics, such news in real life produces only a shocked silence. Families erect a shield of denial almost immediately.

"Rebecca has a deadly form of brain cancer called

primitive neuroectodermal tumor," the neurosurgeon
calmly explained, "a name I know you won't remember.
Bottom line? It cannot be totally removed and we have
no further treatments we can give her because she is a
baby."

"How does a baby get cancer?" asked her grandmother
with an almost cynical tone.

"They're born with it," Dr. Wilson continued. "Cancer
is not uncommon in infants and children."

"Will she be a retard?" sobbed the mother. "Can she
go to a normal school like other children?"

The grandparents shifted uncomfortably in their seats.
Although uneducated, they grasped the reality of the
situation far better than their daughter. Dr. Wilson leaned
close to Mrs. Hobson's face and placed his hand on
her arm.

"Janet," he said in a soft but firm tone as he gazed
directly into her eyes and prepared to drop the bomb,
"Rebecca is not going to school. Rebecca is not going to
have a first birthday party. Rebecca is not leaving this
hospital. Rebecca is going to die. Probably very soon."

"No, no, you're wrong, she's a strong little girl. I
know. She kicked like a mule in my stomach . . ." She
started to cry harder and put her head down on the
room's circular conference table. ". . . She has such
pretty blue eyes . . . Momma, tell me my little girl won't
die."

Rebecca's father sat in the corner opposite to me. He
was hunched over, elbows on knees, smoke trailing from
a cigarette in his left hand. He looked down at the floor
and never spoke. The room fell into an eerie silence
broken only by the occasional soft sobs of Rebecca's
mother.

"We'll talk more later." Dr. Wilson bolted up and started to exit the room, with me close behind. The grandfather followed us out the door while the grandmother stayed behind to comfort her daughter.

"Doc, can I talk with you?"

We closed the conference room door and moved out of earshot down the hall.

"How long does she have?"

"That's difficult to say . . . a few months . . . ," replied Dr. Wilson. "She isn't fully awake yet from surgery, but I'm afraid she may be badly hurt. There is a chance she might have some paralysis or that she might not wake up at all."

"Can we take her home? This is such a long drive and the poor kids don't even have their own car."

"I don't think she'll ever be able to go home. We might transfer her to a hospital in your own state, but since she's on medical assistance now and we began treating her here, they may not pay to take her back. Sounds cruel, I know, but she may be stuck here until she dies."

The old man lowered his head to hide the tears welling in his eyes. "What should we do?"

"Janet may not have formed a truly strong attachment to her child yet. Your daughter is young, she has a lot of time to forget and have another child. My suggestion is that you go home. If you don't come back, we'll understand."

"Don't come back?"

"This baby has no future. Why watch her suffer and die? Go home."

* * *

Rebecca eventually did awaken, but was virtually quadriplegic, with only weak movements of her arms and no movement in her legs. Her swallowing was impaired. She gagged and choked during feeding. Over the ensuing weeks, we inserted a tracheostomy in her neck, a permanent feeding tube into her stomach, and a shunt into her brain.

While Rebecca's mother visited her occasionally, she could never hold her, never feed her. She couldn't bear to watch as the nurses snaked thin tubes into her baby's tracheostomy to suction away the infant formula overflowing into her lungs. Because the tracheostomy entered below the vocal cords, Rebecca could make no sounds. Her gaping mouth cried in ghostly silence.

Finally, the family heeded Dr. Wilson's advice. One day Rebecca's mother stopped coming. Rebecca became the ward of the fifth-floor neuro team. Nurses rotated frequently, to avoid feeling too motherly to the child with no future. Even Dr. Wilson quit making regular rounds on her. She was fed, bathed, and turned. She was given a radio and a ubiquitous Sesame Street mobile to be hung over her crib. Her life became a routine of detached custodial care. She was now adrift in the world, cut free of permanent human bonds, kept at arm's length by those afraid to see children linger. Yet, for some strange reason, I still visited her every day.

Rebecca Hobson responded to the world that had greeted her with an immediate death sentence. She refused to die. At least for a good deal longer than anyone believed possible.

* * *

Months passed. Rebecca developed a round face, dimples, and a full head of curly hair. She smiled and made feeble swats at her mobile. Though she still could not swallow well enough to be free of the feeding tube, nor breathe well enough to be rid of the ventilator, she became a person. The scrawny infant that had frightened me in the ER grew to be a beautiful baby.

Rounds became playtime. I shook a rattle or her stuffed rabbit, the sole gift from her mother, as I listened to the litany of blood work and vital signs registered for the day. I harbored a nagging worry that Rebecca wasn't going to die fast enough, that she was going to grow to be several years old and fully aware of the world before she had to leave it.

Ethicists and cost cutters argue that placing a pillow over her tracheostomy would be the best thing we could do for Rebecca—and for society. Rebecca's hospital costs now topped half a million dollars, a steep price to pay for a baby with a terminal disease. Her death would be brutal, most likely from pneumonia. The ethicists and cost cutters might change their minds, however, if they saw Rebecca. Although imprisoned in a hospital bed, she did not look like she longed for death as she grinned at her rabbit.

Even after I left Children's Hospital to return to the adult service, I would sneak back on my rare quiet nights on call to check on Rebecca. She lasted nine months, a year. She began mouthing words and spending time in a little swinging chair, rocking back and forth with blue plastic oxygen hoses swaying at her side. Her mobile grew faded and worn, her stuffed rabbit stained with pureed food. Her family, although informed of her progress, did not waver in their decision to treat her as already dead.

After my pediatrics rotation was over, I was assigned to the V.A. hospital for six months and lost track of Rebecca, who was now nearing eighteen months of age. One evening, as I was having dinner in the hospital cafeteria, I spied Eric, the current chief resident at Children's. I asked him if Rebecca was still the same.

"No, she's finally started to crump. We think her tumor is recurring."

"Have you scanned her?"

"Why the hell would we do that? Are we going to operate on her again?"

He was right. This terminal slide was what we had all been waiting for since her first operation. Still, the news disappointed me.

I was going to head home, but I instead wandered down to the fifth floor to see Rebecca again. I hadn't seen her for the past six months and was curious to see how she looked, what she could do.

It was evening when I arrived. The floor was quiet. I waved at some familiar faces at the nurses' station and walked quietly down to Rebecca's room at the far end of the hall. I stopped and looked in the window before entering the room.

The mobile was gone and the radio had been replaced by a television set with the volume turned down. The set flickered silent images of a *MASH* episode. The ventilator clicked and hissed a slow rhythm.

Rebecca blankly stared at the screen, her face paler and thinner than I remembered, her lids heavy. Dark circles underlined her sunken eyes, which were beginning to deviate downward again. The left corner of her mouth drooped from increasing facial paralysis, the dimples victim to her resurrected malignancy.

I stepped in front of the bed and peered down at the tiny face, which looked back at me. She paused, then broke into a crooked grin. Her eyes widened and she gleefully twisted her head and struggled to lift her paralyzed arms to embrace me, happy to see one of her few friends.

That moment remains clear and frozen in my mind to this day, more than any other moment in my clinical experience. Although in the years that followed I would take care of thousands of patients, marry, and have two daughters of my own, I may never be as important to anyone as I was to Rebecca that night. As I had gone about my own life, I remained special to this pathetic child imprisoned in her hospital crib.

I spent a long time with Rebecca and her rabbit that night. Ten days later she died. The rabbit was buried with her.

The nurses called me to the neuro floor a month after Rebecca's death. Her family had sent a gift to the floor and they wanted me to see it: a porcelain statue of a laughing girl. At the base of the figurine sat a small brass plaque, inscribed with the words "In memory of Rebecca."

I am not particularly religious. In fact, the birth of children bearing cancers I find difficult to reconcile with a merciful God. Nevertheless, there must be someplace where Rebecca now laughs in the bright sunshine, finally free of her ventilator and gastrostomy.

My facade of surgical psychopathy cracking to pieces,

I left the floor and walked away from Children's Hospital.

Never to return.

11

Nightmares, Past and Future

The first years after receiving my driver's license, I cruised the streets with little regard for the dangers of the road. Protected only by the rusting bodies of cheap used cars, I drove with the confidence of Achilles, afflicted with the youthful delusion of immortality. Until one event penetrated that delusion like the spear which pierced Achilles' human heel.

My revelation came on a snowy Friday evening. I was piloting a 1967 Volkswagen along the expressway leading from the university to my parents' home. Blowing powder barely dusted the roadway, and I believed the traction was normal. That is, until I reached the first overpass and discovered for myself that bridges really *do* freeze before the road surface. I hit the shimmering ice on the overpass going fifty miles an hour. I felt the friction between my worn tires and the glazed road evaporate; the steering wheel became limp in my hands. The car's tail began a slow, clockwise spin; I saw the bridge rails flash by through my windshield as my vehicle turned perpendicular to the road.

The Volkswagen continued to spin and slide. Transiently blinded by the headlights of a truck behind me, I feared being smashed against the concrete abutment. My out-of-control Beetle completed one complete revolution as it exited the bridge, then regained its footing on the warmer asphalt of the roadway before taking off, straight as an arrow. I continued down the expressway at full speed as if nothing had happened.

But something *had* happened. Although I was unhurt and my car undamaged, my outlook on driving could never be the same again. This experience taught me what a dozen Red Highway movies in Driver's Ed did not: how very easy it was to lose control of a car and die. Decades later, I still feel the steering wheel dissolving in my hands as the car slides. One instant in complete command; the next, a terrified passenger thrown upon the mercy of fate for survival.

I had been lucky, learning my lesson and paying no price. If only all lessons were so painless. A Native American proverb states that a child allowed to wander into the campfire learns better than a child told a thousand times to stay away. But this trick fails if that first trip into the fire burns the child to death. On that snowy expressway, I had wandered into the campfire and, by sheer luck, escaped unburned.

Before reaching my surgical adulthood, I would again stray into the inferno of overconfidence. And come perilously close to emotional incineration.

Clipping an intracranial aneurysm tests the full mettle of a neurosurgeon. While this procedure was not the complete measure of our worth—a neurosurgeon who does excellent spine work but can't clip an aneurysm has greater value than one whose proficiencies are the reverse—the residents gauged their machismo using the aneurysm scale. At what point a trainee "did" his first aneurysm, and how many aneurysm notches were carved on his belt when he finished training, were statistics known well throughout the department.

Given the stakes involved, what constituted "doing" an aneurysm spurred hot debate. "Mark said he *did* that anterior communicating artery aneurysm with Gupta, but he didn't dissect it out, he only put the clip on it . . . and that's *easy*." Aneurysms are the bull elephants of our Big Game Club. To put one on your wall, you had to stalk it, stare it in the eyes, and pull the trigger yourself. Letting someone else dissect it out and then ask you to place the clip was like having your hunting guide bludgeon an elephant and then ask you to shoot out the beast's unconscious brain. No fair.

Average on the aneurysm/testosterone scale, I slayed my first (fairly easy) posterior communicating artery aneurysm six months into my senior residency year. In the second six months I clipped several more. The number of my successful cases mounted, each smoother than the last. Although a few patients succumbed to the inevitable complications of brain hemorrhages, I harmed no one with my surgery. My confidence became dangerously inflated. "These aren't so tough," I remarked foolishly to one of the attending surgeons.

"You aren't a neurosurgeon when you clip your first aneurysm," he replied grimly. "You become a neurosurgeon when an aneurysm first blows up in your face . . . have you had that happen yet, son? Has one of those little bastards exploded on you?" I shook my head and he just smiled, the knowing smile of a weathered gunslinger talking with a pompous greenhorn who has yet to feel a bullet pierce him to the bone. The surgeon continued:

"Well, when that first one blows ... let's just say the next one you do won't look quite so easy anymore."

My senior residency year drew to a close. I was five years into the program and slated to start my research time, but due to a sudden change in the schedule, the V.A. beckoned me for three more months of clinical duty. When I took the helm from the previous chief resident, only one patient resided on the V.A. service: Charles Bognar. Charles, in his mid-forties, had seen some action in Vietnam. He had been at the V.A. for less than a day. His diagnosis: subarachnoid hemorrhage.

Charles had experienced the worst headache of his life about forty-eight hours earlier. He said that it had to be bad to achieve the "worst" award; a member of the Woodstock generation, he had known some headaches in his day. The pain overwhelmed him like a "mortar burst" as he made love to his second wife. His admission CT scan showed fresh blood spilling into the left Sylvian fissure, the large cleft between the frontal and temporal lobes—where the mighty middle cerebral artery lives.

The middle cerebral artery, or MCA, is the largest branch of the carotid artery within the head, supplying blood to almost two-thirds of the cerebral hemispheres. In the Sylvian fissure, the thick MCA divides into smaller trunks which exit the fissure and fan out over the brain's surface like nurturing fingers. The junction where the MCA subdivides forms a churning vortex of high-pressure blood—fertile ground for aneurysm formation.

MCA aneurysms can be quite difficult to clip. They hide behind the numerous MCA twigs like plump red birds perched in an arterial cage. These vital branches must be sharply dissected away from the fragile dome before a metal clip can be placed; otherwise they might be inadvertently clipped as well, resulting in a stroke.

Charles the aneurysm was a challenge; Charles the man was unusual. Gregarious to the point of being obnoxious, and given to inappropriate comments, he introduced his wife as the "second Mrs. Bognar . . . and there's sure to be a few more." He loudly gave his definition of a second wife: "someone with real jewels and fake orgasms," much to her evident embarrassment. He also made some very public observations to his fellow ward patients about his wife's sexual gymnastics and how they'd caused a blood vessel to burst in his brain. He was clearly proud that he had married a woman capable of such a feat. His crude statements were accompanied by a sinister, wheezing laughter.

With his long ponytail and sinewy arms covered with obscene tattoos, I could easily fear Charles if I met him in a dark alley. But the ward wasn't a dark alley, and Charles was just one more patient in need of an operation. His angiogram confirmed the presence of a left MCA aneurysm. Surgery would take place on my fourth day at the V.A..

Charles's aneurysm resided in the left side of his brain. To a brain surgeon, there are two cerebral hemispheres: the left one, and the one that isn't the left one. In over 90 percent of right-handed patients, and in the majority of left-handed patients as well, the left hemisphere contains the apparatus for making and comprehending speech, both written and spoken. The right hemisphere does some useful things, too, like helping us get dressed in the morning and giving us an appreciation of Bach (or the ability to compose music, if we're among the few so endowed), but its function is merely desirable. The left hemisphere's function is indispensable. While a total occlusion of the right MCA will leave a patient paralyzed in the left face, arm, and leg, it will spare the intellect and personality. A similar occlusion of the left MCA amputates the patient from humanity and thrusts him forever into a foreign land, where no one will ever speak his language.

A human MCA, the caliber and fortitude of a plastic drinking straw, carries the nectar of life—another example of how our futures hinge upon the puniest of physical structures. Billy Renaldo had discovered how useful the rubbery pencil known as the spinal cord can be. Our coronary arteries, smaller than strands of linguini; our pituitary gland, little more than a raisin of gooey tissue—delicate, but essential to life. To compensate for their fragility, nature coats these organs in heavy armor of bone and muscle. In Mr. Bognar's case, unfortunately, nature could not protect his left MCA from *me*.

Charles went to the operating room as scheduled. The opening was uneventful. I dissected through the scar tissue in the Sylvian fissure with ease, exposing the aneurysm and the MCA branches as they spiraled around the pulsating dome. No need to worry now; I had obtained a good view of the main MCA trunk and was prepared to put a temporary clip should an intraoperative rupture occur. The attending surgeon rested in the lounge, available if I "got into trouble."

Using a microdissector, I worked under the microscope to free the aneurysm from the cage of MCA branches so that I could find the neck and get a clip across it. One MCA branch came away easily, then another. I was almost home!

But as I twisted the aneurysm to get one last look at its

backside, disaster struck. In my compulsiveness to free the MCA branches, I screwed around with the fragile sac one too many times. In a heartbeat, my previously dry operative field turned into a crimson flood. I became paralyzed for a moment, allowing the blood to fill the left side of Charles's head like a basin and spill into my lap. My mind went blank. This can't be happening, it was going so well . . . *what to do, what to do . . . put a fucking suction in there, idiot!* I put the largest suction into the wound and dove down into the gurgling depths in search of the source of the hemorrhage. The aneurysm had blown. But where was the tear? And could it be fixed?

"I have some bleeding up here." My voice quavered as I informed the nurse-anesthetist of the intraoperative rupture. He bolted from the chair.

"How much?"

"A lot."

He pulled the emergency light, summoning help. I screamed for the temporary clip as I relocated the main trunk of the MCA in the bloody maelstrom that swirled within the Sylvian fissure. I placed the clip. The bleeding slowed. The attending surgeon and the anesthesiologist entered the room hurriedly.

"Why didn't you call me?" my staff man thundered over my shoulder, as if I needed more stress.

"It just happened," I whined. "I was just looking around the backside and it blew . . . I have a temporary clip on."

He squinted into the observer side of the microscope.

"Where . . . where is your temporary clip?"

"Here." I used a gold-tipped forceps to point out the clip on the MCA.

"Way down there?! Jesus H. Christ, that's pretty proximal, probably proximal to the striate perforators . . . how long has it been on?"

"A minute, maybe two?"

"Shit! I'll be right in. Meanwhile, try and expose the aneurysm again . . . and the MCA a little further along. Maybe you can slide the temporary clip further downstream."

I placed several long cottonoids into the wound to protect the left brain, which was pulped and swollen. Aspirating the clot, I traced the residual bleeding down to the aneurysm's dome, where, to my horror, I discovered that the dome had been partially torn away from the parent artery. *Bad, very, very bad.* If the tear had been on the dome itself, as had happened with Andy Wood's vertebral aneurysm, I could have easily clipped the aneurysm. Case finished. But a tear at the neck of the dome left a gaping hole in the MCA itself, a hole which was unfixable. A large MCA branch, perhaps the entire MCA, would have to be occluded just to stop the bleeding. I was crushed in a no-win vise: let Charles die on the table, or take out his left MCA and let him die a speechless relic in a nursing home. What would it be?

After a brief scrub, the staff surgeon displaced me from the operator's chair and poked around the anatomy with a suction tip. I cowered in the assistant's chair, awaiting his verdict on the location of the aneurysmal tear, like a small boy awaiting his father's discovery of a picture window shattered by an errant baseball. In an instant, reduced from brain surgeon to child. In the same instant, the life on the OR table had been laid to waste. Charles's vast collection of war stories and dirty jokes dissolved from the dying pink circuitry like a Cheshire cat, leaving only the lifeless Sylvian fissure smiling back at me. The temporary clip, on for over five minutes now, left little hope that the left hemisphere—the precious left hemisphere—would survive.

"There is a big hole in the main trunk of the MCA . . . ," the staff man grumbled with resignation, "and it'll take too long to patch in a superficial temporal artery bypass. I doubt the STA could support the entire MCA territory, anyway. I'll put an encircling clip around the MCA and hope that the vessel stays open. I have my doubts."

He loaded up an encircling clip, designed to wrap around the entire artery in just such a catastrophe, and crushed it around the MCA. The temporary clip was removed. The MCA stopped bleeding, but the branches of the clipped MCA trunk no longer pulsated. In the ensuing minutes, life-giving arteries thrombosed into rods of purple licorice. The staff surgeon shrugged, pulled off his gloves, and yanked down his mask. The act of removing one's mask and breaking sterility before the wound is closed is symbolic, tantamount to pronouncing the patient dead before he has left the operating table.

"Talk to the family, will you, Frank?"

"Yessir. I will do that."

Closing the wound took an eternity, a ridiculous, demeaning exercise, a marathon runner slogging to the finish long after everyone else has gone home. I thought about the second Mrs. Bognar in the waiting room.

I got Charles to the recovery room shortly after noon. He awakened as expected: thrashing his left arm and leg vigorously, but completely motionless in his right arm and leg. When given commands, he simply widened his eyes in a bewildered, doe-in-the-headlights stare. His speech, pure gibberish. The left hemisphere was gone. The head gone, the body would not be far behind.

Retiring to the family waiting room, I asked the few other families present to please leave me alone with Mrs. Bognar. I switched off the blaring TV set and closed the door.

"We . . . we had some bleeding . . . we were forced to put a clip around the main blood vessel of his left brain. . . . He . . . he has had a very large stroke, I'm afraid . . ."

"A stroke? Is he . . . alive?" Her hands began to shake and her eyes filled with tears.

"Yes. Yes, he is alive. But he can't speak or move his right arm or leg. I'm afraid that's . . . permanent."

"Permanent! You mean he's never going to talk again?!"

My eyes looked down. "Yes. Never. He may not even survive."

She began to hyperventilate, then went to a wastebasket and vomited. Collapsing in a heap on the sofa, she buried her ashen face in her hands and began to weep softly.

"Is there anyone I can call for you? Friends? Family?" I knew that Charles had no children from either of his marriages.

"No, leave me alone. You've done enough."

"It was a risk of the procedure . . . it was explained to both of you—"

"Go away."

And go away I did.

The ensuing days were agonizing. Charles spent his waking hours pounding and twisting the sheets with his left hand in purest frustration, yelling "Yaaah . . . yaaah" in vain attempts to make himself understood. Taking care of patients with aphasia, inability to speak, pushes the envelope of difficulty. Rounding on him was torture. The staff surgeon dragged me to see Charles every morning, grimly displaying my mistake to me like the Ghost of Christmas Future tormenting Scrooge with the outcome of his wasted life.

The second Mrs. Bognar confronted me every day with an unrelenting bitterness. True, he had this aneurysm "thing" in his head, but at least he was all right before the operation. Nothing the aneurysm could have done would have been worse than this, in her mind. And she was right. She didn't blame me for the poor outcome of the operation, but she believed her husband had been deceived about the necessity of the operation in the first place. Statistical operations are hard to explain to people. Such operations are rolls of the dice, a gamble that operating carries fewer risks than the disease. Anyone who bets the farm and loses winds up feeling duped.

I sank into a deep depression. Ordinary diversions, such as watching television or eating a meal, lost all meaning. All these things seemed trivial when I recalled my patient writhing in his speech-deprived cocoon. Play tennis? Enjoy myself while Charles suffered? No, I could not.

Sleep became difficult. I had a recurring dream. I was back in the steel mill, where my favorite diversion was watching the great plunger cranes as they pulled hot ingots from the flaming bowels of the furnaces. In my dream, the plunger cranes came equipped with great, glittering aneurysm clips in place of their usual iron jaws. The gaping clip dipped into a glowing furnace for an ingot. As the crane emerged, there were no burning coke embers, but bubbling jets of boiling blood. The bloody, hot ooze sputtered and spewed from the pit's depths, rushing like a river of magma toward me. Clucking workers laughed at me. "Pretender," they teased.

During my waking hours, the final moments before the aneurysm tore replayed in my head over and over again—my own personal Zapruder film—despite my efforts to shut them out. I almost had the goddamned thing clipped! What could I have done differently? If someone else had been doing this case, would things have come out better? Did I play with the dome too long? I simply did not know the answers. Or, worse, perhaps I did.

"Death and doughnuts," our weekly discussion of complications and operative deaths, dispatched the case with little controversy. The aneurysm ripped, the patient stroked out, tough luck. A big yawn for the more experienced surgeons present. A halfhearted discussion ensued on how to handle the situation—whether a bypass operation could or should have been done to supplement flow to the brain, whether barbiturates would have helped, and so on. The complication was chalked up to PD, patient's disease—a bit of hard cheese, those aneurysms. In my mind, I feared a PCP complication: poor choice of physician. I thought seriously about resigning and ending my career as an emergency room doc. Enrico Fermi's admonition came back to me: Be the best or be something else. No room for pretenders here. Had I remembered the great physicist's maxim one patient too late?

Where did Frank the surgical psychopath go? After Andy died, I thought my personality was annealed to steel. I had what it took to face disappointment—or so I believed. Rebecca's illness bothered me deeply, but she was an infant, an aberration. Nobody can watch babies die. But Charles more than bothered me—he tormented me. I was Raskolnikov, the protagonist of *Crime and Punishment*, someone who imagined himself a conscienceless superman until he committed murder and guilt unraveled him. Charles was the first disaster that was my fault and my fault alone. He didn't have an incurable disease, he wasn't ancient and doomed to die of something soon, he didn't succumb to an attending surgeon, he wasn't born with cancer of the brain—he placed the delicate porcelain of life into my hands and I dropped it.

At the death and doughnuts conference, I gazed about the room at the dozen or more staff surgeons present that morning, one hundred years of neurosurgical experience among them. Surely, these were ordinary men? Their learning curves must have devastated dozens upon dozens of lives. Why were they still sane?

Or were they? During his murder trial, Raskolnikov dreamed of a world full of cruel people endowed with such intense belief in their own moral rightness that they never felt the slightest pang of guilt or remorse, even as their world sank into decay. Is that what it would take for me to go on? A blind belief that there was nothing I could have done better, that no one could have achieved a better result than I did on that day?

That is not the way of the scientist, and I still looked at myself as a scientist. Mathematician Jacob Bronowski believed that the credo of science could be found in an Oliver Cromwell utterance: "I beseech you, in the bowels of Christ, think it possible you may be mistaken." To live with my failures, would I have to exit Bronowski's self-critical world and enter Raskolnikov's dreamworld, the megalomaniac's Utopia?

Five days after surgery, Charles's dead left brain swelled and smashed the life out of his brain stem. He was placed on mechanical support. During a tense ten-minute meeting, Charles's wife and I reached an agreement to withdraw his ventilator. On the seventh post-op day, I went into his room and, armed with the ventilator key, accomplished what four years of living with the Viet Cong could not.

My depression did not relent. In my spare time, I returned to the places of my premedicine days—the tennis courts in the park, the undergraduate library, even the grounds surrounding my high school—in hopes that soaking up the ambience of the past would restore me to the person I once was, to the boy who only worried when his forehand sailed long, for whom an overdue book report was the most pressing problem in the world. But I wasn't that boy anymore. I was no longer the bright student capable of anything, the slacker who harvested A's with ease and had the world by the ass. I was now thirty years old, engaged to be married, and possessed of only one way, short of flipping burgers, to make a living. If I bailed out now—changed residencies, went to law school, got an M.B.A.—I risked ending up like William the Registrar, flitting from job to job until I retired, without ever accomplishing anything. Worse, I had no guarantee of being happier or more competent in those fields.

No more second chances. I decided that my random walk through life must end in neurosurgery.

I refused to operate again for weeks after the aneurysm

fiasco, a feat possible on the slow V.A. service. Talking with the attendings about my career doubts would have done little good—a marine boot can't discuss his doubts about the Corps with his drill sergeant. I decided to call Gary in New York.

"Yeah, it's a bitch, isn't it?" I could hear him strike a match in the background. Still smoking.

"That's it?" I grumbled. " 'It's a bitch'—those are your words of wisdom?"

"Who are you feeling sorry for, you or the poor bastard who died?"

"Both of us, I guess."

"I don't think so. Did you go to his funeral, or send flowers or something?"

"Er . . . no."

"So what's bothering you?"

"It wasn't that tough an aneurysm. If Charlie Drake or Thor Sundt or some other full-time aneurysm surgeon had been doing it, Charles would be home screwing his brains out again and working on his next bleed. But it wasn't Drake or Sundt, it was me . . ."

"Let me tell you a story," Gary interrupted. "When I was a third-year resident on neuropathology, I moonlighted at Southland Hospital. One night, some guy drags his buddy in off the street after he has a fight with another guy. We put the buddy on a stretcher and find out that he has a steak knife jammed to the hilt in his right chest. He proceeds to turn to complete shit in front of my eyes and the head ER nurse—one of those iron maidens who has worked in the same place for a zillion years— wheels out this big tray of instruments. 'What's this?' I ask. 'The thoracotomy tray,' she says. The guy needed to have his chest opened all right, but I sure as shit wasn't going to do it. 'Forget it,' I said, 'he came to the wrong man.' He promptly croaked. I felt guilty for a while, real guilty, until I realized two things: one, I didn't plant the fucking shiv into his chest in the first place; and two, if they want a chest surgeon to be sitting in every two-bit ER in the whole world, they had better be prepared to pay him more than forty dollars an hour, which was all they were paying me."

"The take-home lesson of this parable?"

"You didn't make his aneurysm bleed . . . his wife did. And his hypertension, years and years of hypertension—he was no doubt too goddamned busy to see a doctor about it, too. You didn't kill him; you were just asked to step in and prevent him from dying on his own . . . and you couldn't. Yeah, Thor Sundt wasn't there, but Thor Sundt can't do every aneurysm in the country. And I'm sure Thor Sundt has torn a few aneurysms in his lifetime, great as he is—you think he came into this world with a clip applier in his right hand? There will always be people better than you and worse than you. If you worry about not being as good as someone else, why don't you just give up every case right now? Just set up a phone hot line and sit in an office and match people with the very best surgeons in the whole universe. No point in cursing humanity with your own sorry skills, is there? C'mon! Quit feeling sorry for yourself and do the best you can with those who ask for your help. I'm gone just over a year and you start moping over one postoperative death. Yeah, it's a nightmare, but that's neurosurgery. Land of nightmares. There are plenty more nightmares in your future, pal. Remember my index finger: are your coronaries that big?"

"I guess so. How do you do it, Gary? It never looks like you give a shit."

"You have to care about the patients, but not too much. It's unethical to operate on our wives. Why? Because we'd be too likely to choke, to get nervous and fuck up if it's our own family on the chopping block. The very fact that medical ethics forbids treating your immediate family is proof that we shouldn't get so involved with a patient that we are made nervous by the possibility of failure. Patients want us to care about them, but they want us to perform with the nerveless demeanor of someone slicing bologna in a deli at the same time. It's one of those unexplained paradoxes we just accept—you know, like the *Flintstones' Christmas Special*. How do people from a million B.C. celebrate Christmas? Enough bullshit. Clip the aneurysms and take what happens. Don't make me come down there and kick your ass."

Eventually I managed to put Charles behind me. I tossed out my neatly typed resignation letters and halted my searches through the medical want ads. Whether the healing of my psyche came from some maturation process or from the realization that I simply had no other place to go is unclear to me now. Like Raskolnikov in his gulag, I finally acknowledged that psychopathy is not the way to face difficult responsibilities. Some caring is necessary if we are to be the very best surgeons we can be, even if we can't be the best in the universe.

Caring makes the hands shake, but it also makes us dread disaster and work with every fiber of our being to avoid it. Pain, emotional or physical, is the taskmaster of the animal kingdom. The pain of Charles's death taught me a deep respect for the campfire of surgery. I would mind the heat more carefully from now on.

Three months after Charles died, a letter appeared in my university mailbox, a thank-you note from the second Mrs. Bognar. It read simply: "I know now that you only did your best. Thanks for everything."

I was not embarrassed by this thanks, as I had been by the old peach farmer's misguided gratitude so long ago. This was not a generic homage to the magic white cloak. I had indeed done my best; my best just wasn't good enough. I accepted the nightmare of the past and awaited the nightmares of the future.

12

The Wheel of Life

Get up. Shower. Make the coffee. Our lives cycle like planets trapped in their orbits. Each day brings minor variations which cause our individual orbits to wobble a bit—the car breaks down, the school bus is late—but the grand pattern rarely changes. The sun rises and sets. We get up, go to work, retire to bed. The ponderous wheel of life turns inexorably down the road to our uncertain futures.

For some people the stability of life is drudgery. For them, the daily routine carves an intolerable rut, the fixed patterns growing predictable, boring. I, too, once dreaded the ordinary cycles of life. A major motivation for enduring surgical residencies lies in the avoidance of a nine-to-five existence. But as a physician, I learned to pray that my todays will be like my yesterdays, that my orbit remains stable and my wheel of life stays a true course. I pray that I will go home as I have gone home a hundred times in the past, to find my wife and children safe, my parents alive, my house in one piece, my paycheck forthcoming.

I have seen too many patients whose ordinary lives detonated in an instant because of the unexpected: auto accidents, brain hemorrhages, heart attacks. People who awakened to face just one more boring day, and instead found the wheels of their lives careening into the darkness.

There was such a day for Sarah Clarke, age twenty-eight, homemaker, wife of a successful black businessman, and expectant mother of her first child. While preparing dinner in her elegant suburban home, she was startled by an abrupt twitching in her right hand. Her spatula jerked rhythmically out of control. Before she could even become alarmed or cry out, her vision blurred and the room spun violently. She dropped to her knees, then collapsed to the floor in a generalized seizure. The convulsions soon stopped, leaving her stuporous on the floor amid the spilled cake batter and broken cookware. An hour passed before her husband discovered her and had her rushed to the local obstetrical hospital.

At first, no one was sure what had happened. "She just passed out, I think ... maybe from the heat in the kitchen," came the reassuring words of the obstetrician, who further declared the pregnancy in no jeopardy. Such fainting is not uncommon in the first trimester, he observed. Before Sarah could be discharged, however, the seizures returned, first in her right hand and then spreading like a wave to involve her entire body, twisting her trunk in grotesque, violent paroxysms. But this time, the convulsions did not stop until Valium and phenobarbital were given intravenously. The obstetrician, now as alarmed and bewildered as her husband, ordered Sarah transported to the university center—to our neurosurgery service.

As next in line to become chief, I was summoned from my laboratory year to sub for the current chief resident, who had broken his wrist. My first day back on the clinical service, the junior resident paged me to the neuroradiology reading room to help him review a scan on a young black woman. I joined him in the darkened room and we gazed together at the images on the view boxes.

A dark blotch stained her left frontal lobe, an oval hole punched out of the brain tissue. On the enhanced scan, taken after the infusion of intravenous iodine dye, a few areas of white showed up within the ebony hole. Dye cannot enter normal brain tissue, unable to penetrate the chemical shield which protects the delicate brain from all but the most essential nutrients. Portions of the brain where the barrier is destroyed, due to infection, trauma, or tumor, "enhance" by turning white on the CT images.

"Uh-oh," I said, noting the enhancing areas, "looks like trouble for this lady."

"Where? Show me," the junior peered closer.

"There"—I pointed to the small lesion with my reflex hammer—"in the left frontal area. It isn't big, maybe two centimeters, but with some areas of enhancement. Definitely a glial tumor, either astrocytoma or oligo. Could be low-grade, but that enhancement is worrisome. Malignant degeneration may be occurring. . . . Let me guess, she came in with a focal seizure, her hand twitched for a minute and stopped. Am I right? This lesion is too small to give her headaches or weakness, but it's smack in the center of her hand region."

"Close. The seizure did start in the hand, but became generalized. She was found down in her kitchen, woke up, and was taken to Women's Hospital, where they . . ."

"Women's Hospital?"

"Yeah, she's pregnant. First trimester . . . Anyway, to continue, they thought she just fainted, since there were no witnesses, until she started flopping again. Needless to say, the OB guys shit their pants and shipped her here."

"Pregnant. Wonderful. Simply wonderful."

"What do we do now, O mighty acting chief?"

"Put her on Sakren's service."

"He's not on call."

"I know that. But he does the stereotactic biopsies, remember? The only safe approach to this thing is with a needle. An open approach would go right through Broca's area. She'd end up without her speech. No lullabies for junior that way. If there is a junior." The speech area of the left frontal lobe is named for Paul Broca, the nineteenth-century French clinician who first associated left frontal-lobe tumors and aphasia.

"Do you think she'll lose the pregnancy?"

"I don't know . . . probably. While there is nothing about these tumors directly that prevents a normal pregnancy, she may not live six or seven more months without treatment. And I doubt that we could give treatment to a woman who's in her first trimester. She'll need radiotherapy, at least six thousand rads, and you can't shield the fetus from that. At least I don't think so; we'd have to ask the physicists—this problem has never come up before. Chemo might help, but you aren't going to give that to a pregnant woman, either. They don't even let them drink coffee anymore, for Christ's sake. How are we going to blast her with nitrosourea or platinum? She may have to choose between not surviving until her due date and having a therapeutic abortion. There are your choices, ma'am. Have a nice day! I'll go and talk to her. Just think, I gave up dealing with laboratory rats for this."

*   *   *

Sarah was a stunningly beautiful woman, endowed with soft hazel eyes that rode the crests of her high cheekbones. She sat upright in her hospital bed as I entered. Her dapper, well-manicured husband, James, sat in a chair at her side. Although still groggy from the anti-seizure drugs, she managed a smile. The seizure had passed.

"Well, Doctor," she began in a soft, almost apologetic tone, "I guess I'm an epileptic now."

"I prefer to think of it as 'seizure disorder,' and, yes, you do officially have a seizure disorder."

"Why? What's happening to me?"

"Mrs. Clarke, anyone can have a seizure. Some people just have a lower threshold for seizures, that's all. The threshold can be lowered by sleep deprivation, drugs, overexertion . . . or, in your case, a blemish on the brain."

"Blemish? Is that a diplomatic way of saying that I have a brain tumor?"

The comment surprised me. Many patients won't utter the word "tumor," even months after their diagnosis.

"Well, you see . . ." I began to flounder, my carefully planned buildup derailed by the patient's abruptness.

"It's all right." She forced a smile again, sensing my shock. "I heard the technicians mumbling something about a brain tumor . . . they thought I was asleep, but I just had my eyes closed."

I gathered myself. "Yes, you *may* have a brain tumor, but a scan is not diagnostic of anything. It simply suggests what might be there. We will need to obtain a sample of the abnormal tissue and have the pathologists analyze it. . . . It could be an abscess, or . . . or something else altogether." I didn't sound very convincing.

"What else could it be?" The husband's deep baritone pierced the room.

He had outmaneuvered me. I had to tell them the truth. I sat down and pulled my chair closer. "In all honesty, it is almost certainly some form of tumor. Yes, I guess benign infection or some weird stroke are still possibilities, but they would be long shots. Despite that, we still need tissue samples. There are several different types of tumor that occur in the brains of adults, ranging from pretty good to really, really bad."

"So," James continued, "we're talking brain surgery."

"Yes, but a small brain operation. We won't shave very much hair, and it's done under local anesthesia using a special metal frame that is placed on your head. It takes about an hour and is very safe, although all brain surgery carries some risk."

Sarah spoke up. "Why don't you just cut the whole thing out, get rid of it? Won't that make the seizures stop?"

"Mrs. Clarke, your tumor is right here." I pointed to her left temple. "Are you right-handed?" She nodded. "Then your speech center lies just over this 'blemish,' and cutting into that area and trying to remove it all would carry too great a risk to your speech."

They sat in stunned silence for a few minutes, holding each other's hands in a kneading grip that reflected their internalized anxiety. Sarah broke the interlude with her frail voice.

"You do know that I'm pregnant?"

"Thirteen weeks, according to the ER sheet," I replied.

"Will the surgery affect my baby? Or the tumor, or the seizures?"

"The surgery should not affect your child, especially

since it will be done without general anesthetic drugs. The seizures likewise should have little effect, as long as you remain controlled on drugs like phenobarbital that are reasonably safe for the fetus. The tumor . . . well, the tumor is another matter. It all depends upon what it is and what treatments you may need. Some treatments are just not possible in a pregnant woman. I can see no reason why the tumor would harm the fetus, but our therapies most definitely will. You may need a therapeutic abortion."

Sarah turned her eyes toward me and gave me a look of iron conviction. "Jesus is my Savior," she intoned slowly, "and I believe He will let me keep my child. We've been trying for three years to get pregnant. So do your biopsy, but spare me the details of your 'treatments.' I will keep this baby. Please, I don't want to be mean, but leave us alone for a while."

The husband produced a Bible and read silently as I stole away from the room.

Dr. Sakren served as our "stereotactic" specialist. Stereotaxis is the art of placing biopsy needles and other customized tools precisely into the brain's depths, using an awkward, expensive device known as a stereotactic frame. Before the widespread use of stereotactic techniques in the 1980s, tumors situated below the brain's surface were biopsied "freehand," with the surgeon's intuition as the only guide to the tumor's location. The surgeon might cut a large craniotomy flap over the suspected tumor site and take an educated guess as to where the lesion might be, often attempting a dozen or more blind needle aspirates before either achieving a positive diagnosis or abandoning the procedure altogether. "Free-handed" brain-poking carries a high likelihood of missing the tumor completely, and, worse, a significant risk of catastrophic bleeding.

Nowadays, to perform a stereotactic tumor biopsy, the surgeon bolts the aluminum stereotactic frame to the patient's skull under local anesthesia and then takes the patient to the CT scanner. Brain and frame are imaged together so that brain lesions can be cross-referenced with the frame's centimeter markings. Because the frame is held in place by graphite pins drilled into the skull's outer layer of bone, the correlation of the frame's markings with the internal structures of the head remains exact. The position of a brain tumor relative to the metal frame cannot change, even as the patient jostles from operating room to CT scanner and back again. Such accuracy could never be maintained with more civilized means of attaching the frame to the head (with Velcro chin straps, for example).

After the scan, the surgeon chooses a biopsy point on the scanner's video screen, using a light pen, cursor, or computer mouse. In Sarah's case, our target would be one of the enhancing areas within her left frontal lobe. The scanner's onboard computer provides coordinates of the biopsy point relative to the frame's markings. Back in the operating room, a metal arm guides the biopsy needle to the target designated by the computer-generated coor-dinates. Because of the precision of this method, the biopsy requires a scalp incision and skull opening just large enough to admit the biopsy needle (less than half an inch). Since only one or two passes of the needle are needed, the chances of injuring the brain with this method approach nil.

As valuable as stereotaxis has proven, their neuro-surgical peers view biopsy surgeons as wimps—surgeons who do tiny operations because they lack the skill or stomach for "real" brain surgery. Stereotactic surgeons are the field-goal kickers of our specialty: skilled, well paid, and thoroughly indispensable on select occasions, but not true players in the eyes of the more violent members of the team.

I presented the case of Sarah Clarke to Sakren the day after her seizures. He looked at her scan with a squint. "So she wants to keep her baby. Fine, we'll see what happens. But I know the type. 'God wants me to live, He has a special purpose for me.' If God wanted you to live He would not deposit a malignant glioma into your dominant frontal lobe. Personally, I think she should just get an abortion preoperatively and be done with it. What do you think?"

"I think I wouldn't waste my breath asking her to consider an abortion. I can tell you the answer to that question right now."

I had seen the answer in her eyes and heard it in the tone of her voice. Sarah would keep her baby, no matter what. Jesus, and her own iron will, would see to it.

Cancer patients are told to direct anger at their tumors, to "fight" the disease as they would fight some evil, hateful enemy determined to rob them of all that is precious. A useful technique clinically, perhaps, but the emotional colorations should not be taken literally. Cancer is not evil, not the enemy. Cancer is a biological process which has evolved for a very useful purpose: to kill us.

Although we look at ourselves as organisms, we are really societies comprised of trillions of specialized cells—blood cells, nerve cells, muscle cells, gland cells—cells which behave in accordance with communal laws developed for the good of the society. We are like giant hives and our microscopic cells the bees and wasps within.

In any society, certain individuals choose to ignore the societal constraints and march to their own drummers. Likewise, in our own bodies, rogue cells arise which do not respond to the laws regulating their growth. These aberrant cells divide endlessly, creating dysfunctional masses of tissue which compress other organs and commandeer nutrients. The cells escape their normal habitats and metastasize to other parts of the body. Like human miscreants, misbehaving cells have little regard for the society in which they live and will destroy it if given the chance. Indeed, cancer evolved for precisely this reason—to destroy the host.

Cells which grow beyond their normally defined limits are neoplastic; neoplastic cells which invade and destroy tissue, or which detach and spread to other parts of the body, are cancerous. While all cancers are neoplasia, not all neoplasias are cancerous. For example, common warts are neoplastic, but not cancerous.

Most of the scourges of aging arise from neoplasia. In addition to cancers, male prostatism, eye cataracts, degenerative arthritis, and atherosclerosis (hardening of the arteries) result from unchecked proliferation of normal tissues. Even dementing brain illnesses, such as Alzheimer's disease, stem from neoplastic overgrowth of brain cells called astrocytes. As our cellular society grows senescent, neoplastic behavior becomes rampant until our bodies fall, like ancient Rome, into anarchy and ruin. Ubiquitous in the elderly, neoplasia is more a form of planned obsolescence than a disease.

To understand cancer's role in evolution, we must remember that we are built to die. Just as automobiles roll off the assembly line with a predetermined lifespan, the fertilized ovum programs us to decay and perish in an immutable sequence.

The long-term viability of multicellular creatures on this planet demands that each generation enjoy its finite day in the sun and then be thrown from life's stage to make way for a new cast of players. A continuous turnover of organisms, with mixing and mutations of genes occurring in each new generation, gives life flexibility to survive a wide range of climate shifts. There is no biological reason why we could not be immortal. Indeed, we form the tail end of an unbroken chain of protoplasm, five billion years long. However, immortal species would have to stop replicating, else they would smother themselves.

Nature chose not to populate the earth with static, immortal species. To do so would place all of life's genetic eggs in one basket, running the very real risk that some drastic geological event could wipe out all life on earth. To prevent this, the gene pool must be in constant flux, changing at a rate fast enough to keep pace with any environmental perturbations that might arise. Thus, all things must die. Death is not a flaw, a failure of biology, but an essential design feature for constant existence on an inconstant earth. Our downward spiral from youth to old age, like the upward spiral from fertilized ovum to developed infant, is stamped into our genetic code.

The wheel of life: one generation rises like summer wheat, then withers and falls to seed. The wheel turns—

birth, youth, adulthood, parenthood, senescence, death—driven by genetic machinery set in motion so many eons ago. For all its subtleties and infinite beauty, life has but one purpose: to keep the wheel turning. Turning without the least regard for individuals, species, or ecosystems. The destination of the living wheel as it travels through geological time is unknown, perhaps not even important to us. Yes, each generation grows infinitesimally better than the one before it, but better at just a single thing: keeping the wheel moving. The vibrant colors of a bird's plumage, the complexity of a spider's web, the grace of a hunting lioness—all are variations on the single theme of birth, procreation, and death. Adapt, be ready, survive.

For those lucky enough to escape death by predators or accidents, neoplasia in one of its many forms—cancer, dementia, heart attack—will come, a message that all individuals, no matter how worthy they may seem, must give way to the next generation. Regardless of how cautiously we live, our arteries will eventually clog with hardened tissue, our minds grow weak from excessive brain astrocytes, our eyes dim from corneal overgrowths, our organs fill with malignant growths. This is as it should be. Biology doesn't consider these diseases enemies, just as General Motors does not consider rust a flaw. Decay is a necessary process for any business dealing in renewable goods.

We cannot accept our personal dispensability in this scheme. Cancer may be a threat to us individually, but poses no threat to our species. The vast majority of those afflicted by neoplasia are far beyond child-bearing, or even child-rearing, age. Moreover, cancer is a uniquely human affliction. Animals in the wild rarely survive long enough to suffer the neoplastic illnesses of senescence.

The same was true of *homo sapiens* prior to the advent of civilization. A death at eighty from colon cancer would have been a worthy goal for cavemen daily pitted against mammoths and saber-toothed tigers.

Scientists and spiritualists who insist that our bodies harbor some hidden potential to conquer all cancers ignore the trivial effect cancer exerts on our species. Nature does not care if I get cancer, since the wheel of humanity will turn just fine without me. Biology could have easily endowed me with a foolproof method of defeating cancer. And a tire company could make a tire that lasts for a million miles. The awful truth is that neither nature nor a tire company has any motivation to provide unreasonable longevity.

So Sakren, in essence, was right. Whatever entity, divine or earthly, deposits malignant brain tumors into our heads, does so not to test our resolve, to challenge our faith, or to prove our strength, but to make us die. This does not mean that we should not use our intellects to prevent this fate when we can. Such is the very business of the medical arts. Nature discards individuals; surgeons do not. Let nature worry about the species; we must care for individuals one at a time.

At this moment the individual in question (individual plus one-quarter?) was Sarah Clarke. Her biopsy confirmed the presence of a malignant mixed glioma, a small lump of cancerous cells that were to become grains of sand binding up the gears of Sarah's reason. Over time, her mind's clockwork would slowly grind to a halt. Would she let us throw our backs into her wheel of life and push it further along? Would she let us try to extend her life?

* * *

"No way." Linda, the university's chief radiation physicist, shook her head vehemently. We were discussing Sarah. "I've done some preliminary calculations and, even with the most coned-down fields and maximal shielding, the scattered dose to the fetus is unacceptable. Third trimester, maybe, but even then there is the liability issue. There is no way we can deliver any meaningful amount of radiotherapy to this tumor unless the pregnancy is terminated. Period."

"What liability problem is there in treating her in the third trimester?" I asked. "I would think that a fully formed child should be able to tolerate the small amount of radiation that would leak through the abdominal shielding."

"Medically, none. There really isn't even that substantial a risk in the first trimester, either, but try and tell that to a jury. There have been some goofy cases which have produced million-dollar malpractice awards. In Texas, a child is born without a leg and the mother's lawyer successfully argues that an inadvertent occupational exposure to radiation in the ninth month was responsible. You don't have to be too sophisticated in embryology to know that the legs are fully formed in the ninth month of pregnancy and that whatever caused this child to be born with only one leg must have occurred in the first trimester or in the fertilized ovum itself. Yet they bring this little crippled child into the courtroom, sit her in the arms of her crying mother while some expert waves his arms and says that magic word 'radiation,' and the jury gives the kid seven million dollars. Add in the fact that the statute of limitations in children doesn't run out until they are over eighteen, and our department will assume responsibility for the baby Clarke forever if we treat this woman.

If the baby doesn't get accepted into the college of its choice, it can come back and sue us for brain damage. No thanks. If the patient aborts, we'll do it. Otherwise, forget it."

Sakren ran his fingers through his thinning hair. "Goddamned lawyers." A phrase repeated almost daily by neurosurgeons across the country. Lawyers have pretty much determined when we should scan people, when we should operate upon them, and how much better we should make them. To believe that legal issues don't alter the practice of medicine is to know nothing about the practice of medicine in the late twentieth century.

The radiation risk to Sarah's fetus derived as much from the fear of litigation as from tumor biology. Because a fetus is a blank slate, almost any jury award can be conjured up for a pregnancy gone bad. Sarah's unborn child represented a financial burden that no one wished to bear.

Sakren approached the Clarkes about the refusal of the radiation oncologists to give Sarah radiotherapy. "With radiation therapy, you have maybe a one in ten chance of living five years or longer. Not great, but people waste hundreds of dollars a year on much longer odds in the state lottery. Without it, on the other hand, the median survival is only about three to five months, which means you have a 50 percent or greater chance of not carrying the baby to term. I recommend a therapeutic abortion be performed and radiation therapy commenced immediately thereafter."

Sarah's face became serene granite. "I am not a statistic, doctor. I'm not interested in odds. I will not abort my baby."

Sakren's irritation grew. The surgeon turned to her husband. "For God's sake, man, talk to her. If she was my wife, I know what decision I would urge her to make. I wouldn't want to lose her."

James Clarke was unmoved. "Don't talk to us about what we should do or not do 'for God's sake.' My wife has made her decision. She's in the Savior's hands, not yours."

"The Savior's hands didn't do this"—Sakren laid his finger on the small wound on Sarah's left temple—"mine did. And I'm telling you that she needs to have some therapy if she is to have any chance at all of surviving the next six months! I've been in this business for twelve years, and I haven't seen Jesus come and lift one of these things out of a head yet."

"Doctor," Sarah said calmly, "we're telling you that I will not have an abortion. What Jesus does to my head is not important, but what I do to my child is. So you might as well send me home now. I'll have no further therapy."

Sakren frowned. "Frank, get a serum phenobarbital level on Mrs. Clarke today and discharge her on a Decadron taper. If she's forgoing therapy and wants to save her baby, we might as well get her off the steroids, too. Have her come back in one week to have her sutures removed. To residents' clinic."

"Residents' clinic?" I asked.

"Yes, residents' clinic. There is nothing more I can offer her now." Residents' clinic was the dumping ground of patients the staff surgeons no longer wished to follow in their private offices. Although technically overseen by the attendings, the care was relegated to residents.

"But . . ."

"Residents' clinic is fine with us," James said.

Sakren hustled from the room. I cast an embarrassed look at the Clarkes. "He's a little high-strung, I guess."

"Don't make excuses for the man, son," James admonished me. "He has his views, we have ours."

"Do you want to die, Mrs. Clarke?"

"No, I want to have this child." The tears welled in her eyes, the first I had seen. "When you first came in," she continued after a pause, "you said these tumors could be either pretty good or very, very bad. Where does a malignant mixed glioma fit in?"

"Somewhere in between."

"How much in between?"

"Well . . . drop one 'very' in the 'very, very bad' category."

"Fair enough. Fair enough."

Two days after her biopsy, Sarah went home. The race was on. Which would grow faster, fetus or glioma?

Cancers and embryos are kindred spirits, both composed of highly mobile cells dividing at full throttle. A fertilized ovum changes from a single cell to a miniature human body in a matter of weeks. During this period of high-speed construction, cells migrate freely from one region of the embryo to another as complex organs are assembled from amorphous cell clusters. The ability of cancerous cells to metastasize to distant sites is a throwback to the migratory properties of embryonic cells.

The similarity of cancer cells to embryonic cells goes deeper than a simple capacity to migrate. Proteins and hormones produced in fetal tissues suddenly reappear in cancerous tissues of adults. Carcinoembryonic antigen, a protein normally present only in fetal colons, resurfaces in adult colon cancers; a serum test for this protein allows early detection of the disease. Mechanistically, cancer results not from the degeneration of adult tissues into decrepit forms but from their regression into juvenile forms.

Cancer cells relive the heyday of their fetal youths, chucking the staid responsibilities of mature tissues and reverting to the time when they could grow and travel as they pleased. In this way, cancer reflects a symmetry of life. From dust we came and to dust we shall return. The cancer patient ends life as she began it: an amorphous mass of nomadic cells.

While adult tumors arise from differentiated cells lapsing retrograde into prenatal behavior, pediatric tumors arise from islands of embryonic tissue which never matured in the first place. These "Peter Pan" cells won't grow up, acting like embryonic tissue even after birth. Rebecca's PNET was one example of a Peter Pan tumor. Composed of refractory fetal-nerve cells, the PNET endlessly tries to build a new cerebellum—ignorant of the fact that the job has already been completed. The child with a PNET is literally born with brain cancer. The fetal nature of these tumors explains why they are so refractory to treatment. Fetal cells have a mission: to create a child. Their drive to complete this mission is so strong that only killing the patient will stop them. The wheel must turn.

Because of their similarities, cancerous and fetal tissues are both susceptible to anticancer treatments directed against dividing cells. As such, a cancer patient's decision to abort her child lies beyond the scope of ethical debates about pregnancy termination. No one would have blamed Sarah for aborting her child—no one, perhaps, but herself. Whether she based her decision on her religious views regarding abortion or on her desire to see her child before she died, I didn't know.

As her clinic visits progressed, a terrible thing became apparent: the tumor was winning the battle.

I continued to follow Sarah; even residents in the lab have to go to residents' clinic. Two months after her biopsy, a follow-up scan revealed a larger, angrier mass in Sarah's left brain. She grew clumsy with her right hand and made frequent mistakes with her speech and handwriting. Her arithmetic deteriorated to the point where James took over the family finances. Although he had an M.B.A., she had managed the home budget during their five years of marriage and the forced abdication of this job depressed her immensely.

"James won't let me . . . write . . . the gardens," she said haltingly.

"The gardens, Mrs. Clarke?" I asked.

"Yes." She produced a checkbook from her purse. "The gardens . . . these, he won't let me . . . write on them, the gardens, again." The checks were imprinted with a floral pattern.

"He won't let you write checks?"

She nodded vigorously. James stood in the background and never intervened to correct his wife's speech. This may have been denial, or the refusal to embarrass her by publicly acknowledging her obvious decline. Perhaps by living with her he was able to understand her perfectly, and so perceived no need for making translations.

"Do you have headaches?"

"A little time, small . . . knocks," she answered, "my

head . . . uh . . . knocks . . . a little time at the morning once . . . only."

"Uh-huh. How's the baby?"

She smiled, the right corner of her full mouth lagging slightly. "Yes!" The single word spoke volumes.

"Then everything's all right as far as the baby's concerned?"

James spoke. "We were at the obstetrician's last week. Everything's on schedule." I thought of the progressing scan; some things were ahead of schedule.

"The scan shows some worsening edema, Mrs. Clarke. I think we're going to have to put you on some steroids again."

Her smile evaporated.

"How gone worse my head?"

"I think steroids will help. They will help your speech, too."

I prescribed a low dose of Decadron. During the next week, her speech came back to normal, her right arm became fully functional, and her headaches eased. Sarah and James hailed me as a miracle worker. But in my mind, I knew I was dealing with Mephistopheles again. Just as I had bargained with epinephrine to keep B.G with a Teflon heart alive years earlier, I now sold my soul to Decadron. Like epinephrine, steroids are miracle drugs with a price. They give you the result you want now, exacting their pound of flesh later. With epinephrine, the pound of flesh is taken in kidneys and limbs rendered dead from lack of blood. With steroids, the long-term toll is obesity, diabetes, poor wound healing, muscle wasting, and osteoporosis.

Like B.G. McKenna, Sarah left me with no choice. Decadron was the only agent that could be used safely.

Whether it could carry her all the way to her due date in four months remained to be seen.

Months passed. Each week Sarah's speech and headaches worsened, prompting me to go up on her Decadron. The combined effects of her pregnancy and escalating Decadron turned her once lithe body into an obese pear. She became an insulin-dependent diabetic. Her face became bloated and round, her chiseled features obscured. An acne-like rash covered her cheeks and back; her hair became sparse and brittle. The skin on her hands and forearms became thin and bruised, peeling away to form chronic ulcers. She came to her office visits in a wheelchair, her steroid-sapped legs unable to support her expanding girth. I found it difficult to think of her as the person she once was. The complications of her steroid use were profound, more profound than I would have expected from the doses I'd prescribed.

Despite their terrible side effects, the steroids grew less and less effective. Her stuttering speech gave way to "word salads," and, finally, to incomprehensible gibberish. The weakness in her right arm became paralysis. Her pregnant belly grew large as her steroid-atrophied limbs withered. Her body was now being devoured from both ends by two parasites—a cancer and a fetus—each with a mandate to pick her bones clean for their own survival. Obstetricians instruct expectant mothers to take vitamins, but for themselves, not for their unborn children. The fetus will take what it needs and the mother's metabolism will gladly yield it all. Cancer is equally voracious. Sarah was fighting a war on two fronts, and the battle would soon be lost.

I had hoped that the tumor would grow as a spherical

mass and that we would be able to give Sarah radiotherapy once she was into her third trimester. Or that we
would be able to extend her survival by surgical resecting
the tumor once her speech had become so impaired that
surgery could not worsen it further. Unfortunately, the
cancer refused to cooperate. True to its name, the crab
crawled sideways into her cerebral ventricles and spilled
into her CSF. Once in her spinal fluid, malignant cells
floated to her brain stem and spinal cord.

She presented one evening to Women's Hospital with
intractable vomiting. The obstetricians contacted me
immediately, since, at almost eight months of gestation,
she was too far along in her pregnancy for her impending
motherhood to be the likely cause. The OB/GYN resident in the ER gave me an ominous bit of history over
the phone: "Her husband says she just throws up without
warning, without any nausea at all."

I recognized this as "brain stem" vomiting due to the
tumor's invading an area of the brain stem known as the
area postrema—the vomit center. Brain stem vomiting,
unaccompanied as it is by nausea, causes considerable
embarrassment for the patient. She may be feeling fine
one minute and abruptly spewing vomit onto an unsuspecting victim the next. Brain stem vomiting is horrific in
two other respects: It is often impossible to relieve, and
the patient rarely survives for more than a few weeks
after its onset.

The ER resident at Women's asked if we wanted her
transferred to our service. I said no. The time was
approaching when Sarah's baby would have to be
removed, ready or not. Sarah was already where she
needed to be, where she would have asked to be if she

could still speak. Not the best place for her, perhaps, but the best place for her child.

I went to see Sarah on the obstetrics ward. She was awake, but mute. Her right-side paralysis was now complete; it involved the face and leg as well as the arm. A feeding nasogastric tube jutted from her nose. She looked down, slowly rubbing her large abdomen with her left arm as I walked into the room. I approached the bed and she looked up at me with a blank face, then looked down again. Her husband stood up from his chair and motioned me to exit the room with him.

"They are feeding her by tube, but she still vomits a lot," James began. "They tried antinausea drugs, but nothing works. The doctors say that if she keeps vomiting, they will take the baby by C-section this week. She's now about thirty-six weeks and they think it's safer to deliver now than to let the pregnancy go with the persistent vomiting. She's also having a lot of problems with her blood pressure and blood sugars, too. And she may have a phlebitis in her right leg, and they can't treat that. She could have a clot go to her lung at any time and we could lose them both. . . ." He bit his lip and tears filled his eyes.

Inanely, I tried to steer the conversation away from death. "She certainly developed a lot of steroid problems."

James's sullen expression turned sheepish. "Well . . . I have a confession to make. For a few months we doubled the dose of Decadron without telling anyone."

"How could you do that? The prescriptions were for a set number of pills."

"We got more from our family doctor and from the

obstetricians. We told them that we lost your prescriptions and couldn't reach you or Dr. Sakren."

"Why?"

"Sarah wanted to make a series of videotapes for the baby. She taped twenty-one messages—one for each birthday until age eighteen, and special ones for when he graduates from high school and college and for when he gets married."

"He?"

"An ultrasound showed that it was a boy . . . Anyway, to do this, to make all of the tapes, she wanted her speech to be as clear as possible for a month or two until she finished. She wouldn't let me see any of the tapes, so I couldn't help her in any way. She would take fistfuls of pills at a time just so that she could get a few sentences out. Sometimes she would vomit them up. Once we drove to Ohio and went to an ER pretending we were on a trip and needed a refill of steroids, just to get more. Who was going to question us? The tapes are done and in our lawyer's possession. He has instructions to release them at the appropriate times."

"She's a strong lady."

"Too damned strong. I lie awake at night and wonder if we have done the right thing. Lord Jesus, what am I going to do with a baby and without her? What am I going to do? After the baby is delivered, isn't there anything you can do for her? Can't we go ahead with the radiation therapy then?"

"We've discussed this already, Mr. Clarke. The tumor is lining the ventricles and wrapping around the lower brain stem. It may even be in her spine . . . in fact, I would be surprised if it wasn't. Radiotherapy would be cruel at this point."

He nodded, wiping away the few tears that escaped his brimming eyes.

The following day, Sarah had a seizure which lasted for an hour before it could be controlled. That evening, she was taken to the OR.

I saw Sarah one last time, four days after her Cesarean section. She subsisted now on intravenous fluids, and her consciousness waned. As I stood beside her bed, a nurse brought in the five-pound, seven-ounce James Junior, who was the picture of newborn health. The squirming bundle rested in her good arm. Sarah gazed down upon the infant with wide eyes, her mute stare betraying no emotion. After a minute or so, she turned her head away and closed her eyes. I could almost see her will to live exit her body, and I half expected to hear her voice return for one last, Christ-like phrase: "It is finished."

There, in a small room, in a small hospital, in a small city, I witnessed the great wheel of life grind through another revolution of renewal. Parent and offspring had fulfilled their destinies; the tumor would soon fulfill its own.

Did Sarah have enough of her cognition left to appreciate her child during the few days that she had remaining? I didn't know. I hoped that the ultimate irony was not true, that deep within she rejoiced over her victory in the race of a lifetime.

One week after the birth of her son, social services performed a transfer that they hoped never to make again. They moved Sarah from the maternity ward to a cancer hospice. The steroids—the drugs which she had sought like a heroin addict looking for a fix, the drugs which had bought her enough time to make a video

legacy for the son who would not remember her otherwise—were withdrawn.

Years have passed since Sarah's death. I visited her
grave to read the epitaph one last time:

SARAH CLARKE

LOVING WIFE

DEVOTED MOTHER

13

Belonging

I stared at my coagulated corned beef hash and contemplated my first day as the new chief resident of neurological surgery. My white coat freshly starched, my index cards virginal white, and my mind well rested, I knew this state to be temporary, the lull before the storm.

Seven o'clock on a humid July morning. I awaited the arrival of my resident team for our inaugural card rounds. My assigned senior resident was Mark, who had just finished a pathology elective. The new junior resident, Dave, a University of Chicago graduate, came fresh from his internship at Penn. As I drummed my fingers nervously on the table, I felt very alone. Gone were my original mentors, Gary and Eric. I missed their guidance terribly. Although he was in the fourth year of the program, I knew Mark only from death and doughnuts conferences. I had met Dave before, when I escorted him on his residency interview, but that was over two years earlier. The intern (like all interns) was a complete unknown. A baby-faced lad named Bob, who wanted to be an orthopedic surgeon when he grew up, filled the position this month. Ugh! A team of virtual strangers assembled to help me face the lightning.

The success of a chief rests with the resident team.

When in full swing, the university service carries twenty or thirty patients on the floors, another six on the porch, ten in the intensive care units, and a dozen or more followed as consults. Our surgical schedule could total nine or ten craniotomies and a dozen spine cases in a day, not counting traumas and other emergencies. The workload had increased by over 50 percent since my junior residency year, while the number of residents assigned to the university service remained the same. By way of comparison, a chief resident in the early 1960s faced an average inpatient census of *eight*. The great Cushing did just over two thousand brain operations in his career. Our program did that number in a year. Like other surgical subspecialties, neurosurgery grew exponentially in the 1970s.

I could not know everything that happened on the service, but this didn't stop the faculty from expecting their chief to be omniscient. I had to rely upon the lower-level house staff for information.

The chief resident straddles two worlds. To the younger residents, the chief is just one more taskmaster who decides when they will take call, how many spinal taps they will perform, and what operative cases they are "ready" to do. To the attending staff, the chief stays a scut dog, a lackey who dances to their every whim. The chief resident is a sergeant in the surgical military, friend to neither enlisted man nor officer, endowed with great responsibilities but given little true authority. Despite the abuse heaped upon the chief by the attending surgeons, I had to stay cheerful and cooperative at all times ("Eat shit as if it's your favorite dish," in Gary-speak). Being less than a year from a staff job myself, I could ill afford to mistreat the staff surgeons—indispensable sources of job leads and reference letters.

At 7:15, Mark, Dave, and Bob made their way to the table with trays full of food. The charge nurse for the neuro unit joined us.

"Sooo glad to see everybody is right on time!" I moaned, glancing at my watch. "Since the boss just told me the new rule—the residents must be in their respective OR's by twenty after seven—that leaves us with five whole minutes to cover twenty-two patients. Eat fast, gentlemen."

The intern went first. In quick fashion, I found myself bitching at him about bowel movements, post-op headaches, and sleeping patients in the same imperious tone Carl had used in my third year of medical school. It was a weird feeling. Years later, I had a similar feeling on a driving trip. I turned to my bickering daughters and threatened to stop the car in the middle of the turnpike if they didn't keep quiet. In that instant, I became my father. Likewise, I now became Carl, Maggie, Gary, and every other chief resident I had ever known. The wheel turns. Each generation yields to the next, leaving behind some legacy. In six years, Dave would be sitting in this same spot, sounding just like me.

We sprinted through the patient problems and headed for the operating rooms—fifteen minutes late. Needless to say, the boss was furious. So started the worst year of my life.

"Goddamn it, Vertosick, is this the same case?" The boss growled at me from outside the OR as he held the swinging door open with his right foot. In the vernacular of surgeons, asking the operator if he or she is doing the "same case" is an insult, an implication that a better surgeon would have progressed to a new patient given the same amount of time.

"Yes sir, it most certainly is the very same case. I had some bleeding from the sigmoid sinus, but it's stopped now . . . I'll be ready to open the dura in another ten minutes."

"I sure hope so. We have a cervical disc to do in this room next and I have a medical executive committee meeting at three, so look sharp."

So it went—day in, day out, week in, week out. Staff surgeons beating me constantly. "Same case?" "I have to be somewhere at three . . ." "Just what the fuck do you think you are doing?" "STAY AWAY FROM THE OPTIC NERVE PLEASE."

I ate irregularly and my weight dropped twenty pounds. I feared exiting the hospital, terrified that I would not be there when a patient crumped or a trauma rolled in. Because the chief resident is not supposed to take "in-house" call, the surgical administration assigned me no bed in the hospital—even though I spent more nights there than the junior residents. I wandered the hospital in the darkness, like a homeless person in search of someplace warm and soft to sleep. A transplant fellow habitually occupied the sofa in the surgeons' lounge, so I had to be resourceful. If the ward wasn't full, I used a patient room. Otherwise, I sacked out on the residents' pool table. Slate can be quite comfortable when you haven't slept for thirty-six hours.

I never had the nerve to sleep in one of the OR's, although previous chiefs often resorted to this. Given the aggressiveness of our transplantation team, I worried that I would wake up minus my liver.

*   *   *

Our transplant service carried a very high profile and consumed the lion's share of our health center's OR time and other resources. Their star status imbued the transplant surgeons with the sort of smarmy, menacing charm exuded by *bandidos* in old westerns. During my residency years, transplant stories became daily fare on the local television news programs, making the senior transplant surgeons into celebrities and hailing every permutation of donor, recipient, organ, and disease as a medical landmark. ("Girl becomes first Asian to receive an African-American lung for the treatment of pulmonary hypertension . . . film at eleven!") Our center was, and still is, a transplant center of unequaled excellence, but I grew irritated by the news media's perception that saving a life with an organ transplant is more admirable than saving a life by draining a subdural hematoma or reversing a diabetic coma. When one popular liver-transplant recipient, who had been tracked for years by local journalists, died suddenly, the mayor declared a day of mourning. A tragic death, yes, but aren't they all? When would the city declare a Sarah Clarke day?

Heart and liver transplants are indeed heroic affairs, requiring consummate skill to perform and extraordinary fortitude to undergo. But when viewed from a national health-care perspective, such transplants equal zero-sum games: a life saved is a life lost. Our city coaxed people into signing donor cards, although no one really wants to think about ending up young, healthy, and brain dead. Transplant programs survive on a constant diet of good-looking cadavers—people in the prime of their lives with brains extinguished by senseless catastrophe. In adults, our donor supply flowed from auto accidents and gunshot wounds; in children, donors were victims of parental shakings and beatings. By definition, a donor organ flows from some tragic and eminently preventable event.

Although transplant patients now do quite well, few recipients survive as long as the donor would have had he dodged a bullet or missed a telephone pole and kept his own organs a while longer. I support organ donation wholeheartedly—it makes the most of a bad situation—but we shouldn't lose sight of a larger objective: preventing people from *becoming* donors in the first place.

The neurosurgery service suffered frequent contact with the transplant surgeons. Their potential donors were usually our patients first. Outside hospitals even transferred brain-dead patients to our neuro unit just to be evaluated as donors, a practice which irked us no end. Not only did this practice tie up our beds, but our junior residents had to do histories and physical exams, draw blood work, and manage IV fluids on living corpses—typically in the middle of the night—to spare the transplant fellows such trivialities.

Before the advent of sophisticated organ-procurement networks and transplant foundations, the task of approaching relatives for permission to harvest the organs fell to the donor's attending physicians (and then, in turn, to the neurosurgery resident on call). Occasionally, we were surprised to learn that the family hadn't even been told of the patient's "legal" death. Outside physicians often sidestepped the issue, telling relatives that their dead loved ones were being transferred to the university for further "evaluation"—a true, if not completely honest, statement.

On occasion, we solicited permission for organ donation from the person who made the donor brain-dead in the first place. One of our residents had to call the county jail and obtain permission from the donor's husband— minutes after the man had been arraigned for shooting her in the brain. The suspect later claimed that he wasn't responsible for his wife's death—the transplant surgeons were. He was convicted of murder.

The donor business brought other surprises. A young brain-tumor victim was flown in from New York for immediate donation to a dying liver recipient. The recipient was already in the OR holding area, prepped and ready to go. The transplant team had been summoned. Preliminary tissue and blood typing revealed an excellent match. One teeny problem: the donor wasn't brain dead yet. The junior resident, Dave, called me at home and told me that the patient decerebrated to painful stimuli.

Brain death means the loss of all cerebral and brain stem function as determined by neurological examination. Although ancillary testing, such as EEG (electroencephalograms, a measure of electrical brain activity), can be used, the diagnosis of brain death remains clinical. A brain-dead patient cannot exhibit meaningful movement of the extremities, respiratory motions, response to pain, pupillary response to light, or a gag reflex. Decerebration, the rigid extension of all four limbs to pain, requires a living brain stem and invalidates the diagnosis of brain death.

I told Dave to scan the patient immediately and rushed from home to see this Lazarus. When I arrived, the prospective donor was back in the neuro unit, surrounded by a jittery team of transplant fellows. Dave stood by the X-ray view box looking at the CT scan.

"This 'donor' has a big cerebellar tumor," said Dave

under his breath, "and we might be able to help him, but the vultures are here." He cast a look over his shoulder. Our nickname for the transplant surgeons derived from their uncanny ability to smell impending brain death. They circled the ICU on a daily basis.

"Screw the vultures, I'll deal with them . . . Just take him downstairs and we'll take this thing out. What Massachusetts General Hospital did he come from, anyway?"

"I don't remember. Some place in outer nowheresville . . . they told the family he had a cancerous tumor and was as good as dead. Of course, since they heard so many nice things about transplants from the news, they wanted to give his organs. Nice gesture, but a bit premature."

I approached the transplant team. "Sorry, gentlemen, but, to paraphrase Mark Twain, the reports of this man's demise have been greatly exaggerated. We get to keep him. Maybe next time."

"Horseshit," a transplant fellow spat with venom. "Look at him, he's decerebrate, he'll be dead soon. We'll wait an hour or so and stop back."

"What neurosurgery residency did you train in, my learned friend? Decerebration from posterior fossa lesions isn't as ominous as you think. Our New York friend could be eating eggs for breakfast by tomorrow."

"Eating osmolyte through an NG tube, you mean. I know a brain-dead guy when I see one, and I have a lady in hepatic failure downstairs."

"Is this a Monty Python skit or something? He isn't dead yet and you can't have him. So kiss off."

The large group flowed from the room. We removed the man's tumor that night and he walked out of the hospital a week later. The donor pool was reduced by one, but this particular patient didn't seem to mind. Two years passed before his tumor claimed him for real.

Clang! What sounds worse than a phone ringing in the middle of the night? When the intern took in-house call, it wasn't worth going to bed at all. I pulled the phone receiver to my ear. Bob, the orthopedic wannabe, chattered excitedly.

"It's a gunshot wound! Right between the eyes! What'll I do? Should I scan the patient or take her right to the OR?"

"Slow down, Bob. Where are the entrance and exit wounds?"

"The entrance is right between the eyes, like I said. About a centimeter hole just above the bridge of the nose. The exit wound is in the occiput, but a lot of hair and blood's matted there and I can't be sure exactly where the exit is . . . I'm afraid to look too close . . ."

"Relax. I wouldn't want you to puke in the wound or anything. Is the patient intubated?"

"No. She's awake, actually."

"How's that again?"

"She wants a cup of coffee . . . should we let her drink anything if she's going to the OR?"

"Let me try this again. She has a bullet enter between her eyes and exit at the back of her head and she wants a cup of coffee? Is that right?"

"Yeah. She was unconscious when she came in, but woke right up! Weird, don't you think?"

"Call the CT people in. I'm coming in, too. I have to see this. In the meantime, ask her if she wants cream and sugar. Pour one for me, too. Extra sweet. See ya."

I dressed hurriedly. This lady couldn't stay conscious

for long, I thought. Surely the bullet must have clipped a large venous sinus. Even if it didn't, her brain had to swell soon. When I arrived, the victim was still in the ER, awaiting her CT scan—not in a patient exam room, but sitting in the waiting room watching the late movie, her head wrapped with a bloodied Kerlix gauze. A city policewoman sat beside her.

"Are you the woman who was shot?" I asked.

"Uh-huh," she replied trancelike, her attention still focused upon the TV.

"Could you come with me please?" I crooked my finger at her and motioned to the ER's metal doors. She cast me an irritated glance, but obeyed. Back in an examination room, she explained what happened.

"My boyfriend was a little drunk and got real mad, you know, like really, really pissed off, so he shot me. I think I passed out right after it happened. I know he didn't mean it . . . Do you think, you know, I could go back to him tonight? They say I can't." She motioned to the sphinxlike officer who had followed us into the room. "I know that he truly loves me. He didn't mean it, I know he didn't."

The wounds were as Bob had described them. I examined the back of her head, parting the thick brown hair until I saw a jagged exit wound. As I was rummaging around, a nearly pristine bullet fell onto the gurney and was quickly retrieved by the policewoman and turned over to a homicide detective waiting outside. Neither wound was bleeding, and there was no sign of brain tissue or spinal fluid. Her neurological exam was normal. Why was this woman still alive?

The CT scan provided the answer. The bullet had fractured the frontal bone, but had not injured the brain.

Between the scalp and skull at the top of her head was a mixture of blood and air which traced from the entrance wound to the exit wound. The bullet had hit the frontal bone and deflected upward, circling over the skull and under the scalp like a roulette ball before blasting out the back of the head. The woman's skull was unusually thick, a congenital abnormality which had saved her life. She had sustained the handgun equivalent of comedian Steve Martin's "arrow through the head" sight gag.

As amazing as her injury was, her attitude surpassed it. She held no animosity whatsoever toward a man who had jammed his revolver between her eyes and pulled the trigger. After all, he "missed," didn't he? She refused to believe that he had done anything wrong, save for drinking too much and losing his temper.

The skull does a marvelous job of shielding the brain. A middle-aged Protestant minister with intractable depression decided that he couldn't wait until his appointed date with destiny to meet his Maker. He borrowed a friend's .22 caliber revolver and, placing it against his right temple, blasted himself senseless. The paramedics, believing him mortally wounded, transferred him to the hospital without intubating his trachea. He arrived in our ER still unconscious, a serene look upon his craggy face.

Because his vital signs were normal and his pupils reactive to light, I ordered a plain skull film immediately. The X ray confirmed my suspicions: the small bullet had lodged in his "pterion," a hard ridge of bone about two inches in front of the external ear canal. The projectile had failed to enter the brain. The impact of the bullet had struck the minister like a heavyweight uppercut, temporarily rendering him unconscious, but unhurt.

I looked into his face closely as he regained consciousness, curious to see the reaction of a man who believed he was opening his eyes in Paradise. The eyelids fluttered, the eyes squinted into the fluorescent light.

"Is . . . is this heaven or hell?"

I overcame my almost irresistible urge to play some form of practical joke, like lighting a match in his face. "To tell you the truth, Reverend, it's the emergency room. Although it can be hellish at times, I'll admit."

He sobbed uncontrollably, covering his face with his hands. "Oh God, I'm so ashamed . . . so ashamed. I can't even kill myself. . . ." Such a profound and desperate act thwarted by an inch of bone. The irony. Betrayed by the Maker's own blueprint. I said nothing else, leaving him to his inner torment.

He was given a tetanus shot and transferred to psychiatry. I never saw him again.

Monday morning. Residents' clinic. Failed-back patients and neck injuries littered the schedule. One patient caught my eye, however: Florence Janeway. Diagnosis: meningioma.

Three coverings wrap the brain: the dura mater, arachnoid, and pia mater. These wrappings are known collectively as the meninges. When meninges become infected with bacteria, meningitis results. A tumor of the meninges goes by the name of meningioma.

Meningiomas, nearly always benign, arise from the outer surface of the skull, not the brain, and are removed fairly easily. They may take years, even decades, to reach a symptomatic size, given their slow growth rate.

Neurosurgeons enjoy meningiomas. So much so that Mrs. Janeway's appearance in residents' clinic was enigmatic. Why hadn't a staff surgeon snapped this up? It couldn't be because of her insurance status. The staff would *pay* patients for the pleasure of rolling out their big, juicy tumors. Dave had already seen the woman.

"Dave, what's a meningioma doing in our clinic?"

"Oh, you mean Janeway? She's a pretzel lady. Had a history of depression, couple suicide attempts. Now she has Alzheimer's disease and lives in Allison Manor Nursing Home."

"How did they figure out she had a meningioma?"

"One of the aides at the home noticed a lump on the back of her head while combing her hair. They sent her for a scan. I have it in the office."

"How old is she?"

"Sixty-seven."

We returned to the office. Dave flipped the scans onto the view box. Mrs. Janeway didn't have just any meningioma, she had the mother of all meningiomas. A huge white ball occupied a third of her head. Meningiomas induce thickening of the skull, hence the "bump" noticed by the nursing-home aide.

When I saw her, I realized why Dave had called her a "pretzel lady." Muscle contractures distorted her limbs. Her blank face stared into space. She said a few words and followed simple commands, but she certainly looked like someone suffering with Alzheimer's disease.

"What are we supposed to do with her?" Dave asked.

"How do they know she has Alzheimer's?"

"Well . . . look at her!"

"How do we know this isn't from her tumor?"

"I guess we don't."

"Someone gave her the diagnosis of incurable dementia without doing a head scan?"

Dave rummaged through her thick outpatient chart. "That's what it looks like."

I thought for a moment. "The horse is out of the barn, I'm afraid, tumor or no tumor."

"The horse isn't just out of the barn," commented Dave as he looked down at the twisted little frame on the exam table, "it's at the lake getting a drink of water."

"Send her back. Tell the nursing home 'No, thanks.' "

I finished seeing patients and returned to the wards.

But Mrs. Janeway didn't leave my mind that night. Or the next day. Was her dementia irreversible? Sixty-seven isn't old, and her health was good. I called her oldest daughter.

"Mom's been bad for two years. The depression came on about three years ago, but the memory loss and incontinence began two years ago. The last six months, she hasn't recognized me or my sisters at all."

"Three years ago, what was she like?"

"Mom ran an insurance office for thirty years. Sharp as a tack. Then she started having trouble with arithmetic and had to quit work. That was ... hmmm ... about 1976."

I explained the situation, described the tumor, and detailed the risks of surgery—considerable, given the large size of the mass and the fact that it pressed on her left brain. She listened politely, but declined surgery.

But the issue gnawed at her as much as me, and I received a phone call the next morning. The three children had talked (Mrs. Janeway was a widow). They wanted surgery. As I suspected, neither they nor I could live with the slightest possibility that a working brain had been abandoned to the mercy of a benign tumor. I scheduled the craniotomy for the following week.

I requested the boss's help—I needed his thirty years of experience.

It was a bloody affair. We reflected the thickened bone from the bulging mass beneath and released a torrent of bleeding. I incised the dura, located the plane separating brain from meningioma, and began pulling the mass out of her head. My slow technique, however, could not keep up with the bleeding.

"This will take forever," I moaned.

"We need to get it out fast," observed the boss calmly. "We're losing about two hundred cc's of blood every fifteen minutes." He looked over the anesthesia screen and spoke to the anesthesiologist. "Can you folks keep up?"

"Possibly, but we don't want to get into big fluid shifts in her."

The boss looked back at me with a gleam in his eyes. "Frank, get some cotton balls and have your bipolar ready. We're going to yank this thing the old-fashioned way. Quick. Are you ready?" I nodded. "Then put a great big nylon stitch through the dura over the tumor . . . here . . . that's it . . . Now I'll put my finger here . . . OK, PULL!"

I pulled the suture as the boss swept his large index finger beneath the tumor. The red baseball levitated from the wound as the chairman advanced his finger deeper. The bleeding increased. I jammed cotton balls between the tumor and the brain with my right hand, my left hand providing traction on the tumor stitch. As he delivered the tumor from the depths, the boss inserted another finger, then another, until Mrs. Janeway's head swallowed his hand.

The anesthesiologist grew nervous. "We're getting hypotension here."

"Fix it," the boss yelled without looking up, "that's what they pay you for. Come on, Frank, buzz that artery . . . there. Keep working, we're almost home."

Finally, the great mass slithered out of the skull and dangled on a shred of uncut dura mater. A snip of the scissors and the tumor dropped into a steel pan. Stopping the bleeding took an hour longer. When everything was dry and the patient stable, we could at last see the horrible brain deformation left behind. The meningioma had flattened the left hemisphere into a pancake, and our surgery had chewed up the cortex terribly; I doubted that the brain would recover.

Nevertheless, the boss looked pleased.

"Nice work. That was a monster." He shook my hand before pulling off his gloves. "You're really one of us now."

I still see Mrs. Janeway once a year. She comes to the office in her smart business suit and tells me about the latest Buick she drives. Her legs remain stiff, although the orthopedic procedures to release her contractures worked wonders. Her daughters claim she is every ounce the woman she was fifteen years ago.

In my career, Mrs. Janeway was truly a landmark case. If I never accomplish another thing in my life, I will go to my grave satisfied. I will not walk on the moon, or win the Nobel Prize, or live in the White House. But the rare privilege of snatching someone from a nursing home and giving back her mind, her life, her family . . . I wouldn't trade that for the world.

Despite the occasional Mrs. Janeways, chief residency ground me down. Constant exposure to gunshot wounds, brain-dead donors, harried interns, pompous surgeons, patients in pain, and hospital-grade corned beef took its toll. My enthusiasm for the job waned. Some days I no longer cared who lived and who died. I just wanted to be done, to have my life back, to see my wife and baby. Like Humphrey Bogart in *The African Queen*, all I could do was climb back into the leech-ridden waters and keep pulling my boat toward the open sea.

My residency ended at last, and with little fanfare, I entered practice. "One of them." Big deal. Overdosed on surgery my final year, I felt little joy for my new profession those first months as an official neurosurgeon. My training finished, I reflected upon my career choice.

We are all slaves to chaos—chaos in the scientific sense. Chaos theory predicts that the outcome of a chaotic process depends upon minuscule variations in the "initial conditions." Example: a billiard ball rolling off the hood of a car. When placed in one spot, it rolls one way; placed one millimeter to the right or left of that spot, it rolls in a different direction altogether. Where the ball ends up depends entirely upon where we place it initially.

The impact of the initial conditions has been named the "butterfly effect," since, in the chaotic theory of weather, the beating of a butterfly's wings in Asia can cause a hurricane in the southern Atlantic months later. Our lives evolve from our own butterfly effects. The tiniest perturbations in our youths, our "initial conditions," generate profound alterations in our later lives. In my case, I had wanted to be a computer scientist, but no openings in my freshman computer-science courses existed. If I had jumped one or two places ahead in the registration line, I would have made it into freshman comp sci and never become a physician. What delayed my arrival at the registration office? I don't remember—stopping for a hamburger, maybe, or speaking to a friend—but whatever this long-forgotten event was, it changed my life. If I could have taken cardiac surgery, as I had wanted, I would probably be one of the "best in the chest" now, and not a brain surgeon.

The butterfly effect: a conversation here, a missed flight there . . . happenings which redirect the rivers of our lives. After buffeting about in the chaotic currents, I feared that I had been cast onto a distant shore, a place where I didn't belong.

Three months into my new practice, a seventy-year-old widow named Grace Catalano came to my office, pushed along in a wheelchair by her burly son. She had suffered from back and leg pains for years. The pain worsened with prolonged standing and walking. In fact, she could now barely walk at all, save for the few steps from bed to wheelchair.

"Oh, Doctor, you are my last hope. I have arthritis so bad in my back and legs, so bad, I can't go from here to the door. Now the pain bothers me even at night, even when I'm off my feet. They have me on narcotic pills. My family doctor says that it's just arthritis and I have to live with it, but a neighbor says that maybe it's a ruptured disc or something. I'm afraid of surgery, Doctor, but I'll do anything to get rid of this. Anything. I have two granddaughters—twins—they are four years old now and they want to know why their grandmama never walks with them or takes them to movies. . . ." She began to wipe her tears away.

I examined her, but detected neither weakness nor numbness to confirm her spinal problem. Her story sounded like lumbar stenosis, arthritic narrowing of the lower spine. Lumbar stenosis results from deposition of bone spurs and thickened ligaments in the lower verte-brae. The spinal canal, which conveys the nerves to the legs, narrows during stenosis. A napkin-ring constriction of the nerves forms, with chronic leg pain as a result. The disease occurs in the elderly and still goes largely unrec-ognized, the leg pains and shuffling gait attributed to incurable arthritic deterioration of the spine, or to old age. Fortunately, even in the advanced stages the condi-tion responds well to surgery, the overgrown bone and ligaments safely trimmed away.

I ordered a myelogram, which verified severe nar-rowing between her fourth and fifth lumbar vertebrae, at the base of the spine. I performed a laminectomy and decompressed her spine uneventfully, but she left the hospital in her wheelchair. Transferred to a rehabilitation center, she didn't return to see me until months later.

Glancing at my office schedule one day, I noticed that Grace Catalano topped the list. When I entered the exam room, however, I saw her son, not Grace, seated on the exam table.

"Where's your mother? Is she all right?"

"Mama didn't want to come in. She wants you to go out in the waiting room." I agreed.

There, erect as a young sapling, stood Grace Catalano, flanked by two raven-haired little girls.

"Watch," she said. Her son swung open the waiting-room door and Grace waddled into the long corridor outside, a granddaughter on each hand. She strolled easily for twenty yards, then slowly turned around and returned. We looked at each other with matching grins.

Yes indeed, if it was easy, everyone would do it. I checked her wound, made some small-talk and said goodbye.

She strode back into the corridor, out of my life and back into her own, her precious grandchildren at her side. Mrs. Catalano was where she belonged.

And so was I.

Look for these true stories of the dangers,
pressures, and triumphs of life on
the front lines of medicine brought to you by
The Ballantine Publishing Group.
Available in bookstores everywhere.

BAG BALM
AND DUCT TAPE
Tales of a Vermont Doctor
by Beach Conger, M.D.

When young Dr. Beach Conger left Berkeley and
accepted a hospital appointment in rural
Vermont, he envisioned living out the rest of his
days splitting wood, healing the sick, and being
adored as a kindly country doctor. What he did
not know about was the education he would
receive from his new patients in the art of country doctoring. BAG BALM AND DUCT TAPE
is an engaging chronicle of the re-making of a
doctor.

Published by Fawcett Books.
Available in bookstores everywhere.

DOC SUSIE
The True Story of a Country Physician in the Colorado Rockies
by Virginia Cornell

In 1907, Doc Susie came to Fraser, Colorado, with a bad case of tuberculosis and a broken heart. But she soon forgot about all that and led a remarkable life as a healer. Here is the amazing and inspiring story of a woman who defied her times and her fears to help those who needed her.

DOC
Then and Now with a Montana Physician
by R. E. Losee

In 1949, Ron Losee, a Yale Medical School graduate, settled in a log cabin in Ennis, Montana, and set up his practice. Doc Losee shares nearly half a century of dedicated doctoring, evoking the rich flavor of Montana and the sometimes dramatic, sometimes comic dilemmas that embroider the life of the country doctor.

Published by Ivy Books.
Available in bookstores everywhere.

A DOCTOR'S STORY
From City Surgeon to Country "Doc"
by William T. Close, M.D.
With a foreword by Glenn Close

William T. Close has lived a life in medicine. His unique odyssey took him from surgery in the inner city to extraordinary work in the heart of Africa to a rural practice in the wide open spaces of Wyoming. Here is a vividly personal account of the making of a doctor and a man of great insight and courage.

A FAMILY OF DOCTORS
by David Hellerstein, M.D.

Dr. David Hellerstein traces five generations of American medicine, from the Civil War up to today, as illustrated by the hardships and triumphs of his unforgettable family. Poignant and deeply moving, this is a chronicle of American medicine unlike any other.

Published by Ivy Books.
Available in bookstores everywhere.

A WOMAN IN RESIDENCE
by Michelle Harrison, M.D.

Based on the diaries Dr. Harrison kept during her residency in OB/GYN, here is the intense inner life of a large hospital in all its complexity. Laid bare are the pressures between patient care and hospital convenience, the excitement of new and successful procedures, and the struggles of over-burdened doctors to find time for yet another patient. You will not soon forget this portrait of a medical community as you have never seen it before.

Published by Fawcett Books.
Available in bookstores everywhere.